RESTORATIVE YOGA

Restful Poses to...

Cradle the Body

Comfort the Heart

Calm the Mind

Nancy Hodge Long, MA. HITA, RYT

ISBN: 978-0-9721003-5-9

DEDICATION

This book is dedicated to my husband, Michael, who never doubted, and patiently reminded me, I could accomplish this. My biggest supporter and advocate, he is also my primary editor, providing countless critiques of sentence structure and wording to help bring clarity and conciseness. The result of his careful eye and endless probing is a book accessible to everyone, especially those who have never tried Yoga.

ACKNOWLEDGMENTS

In the creation of any book, there are numerous people to acknowledge and thank. It is truly a team effort.

I bow in deep gratitude to my teachers, and their teachers and the hundreds of Yoga masters throughout history who have been beacons of light for each of us as we find our way.

I am overwhelmed by the encouragement from my Yoga students and friends who share the love of Yoga and inspired me to write down the practices I share with them.

I want to thank the women in my writers' group who supported me in every phase of this project.

Many thanks to my sister, Tracy, who diligently read and reread my draft, providing helpful comments.

In addition, I am grateful to Sierra Myers, photographer and cover designer, for her creative eye, focused effort, and tireless work preparing the photos for this book.

These acknowledgements would not be complete without honoring the memory of Payton, our Golden Retriever, whose unconditional love and loyalty provided the perfect space to nourish my dreams and fulfill my deepest heart's desire.

CONTENTS

INTRODUCTION

When I found Yoga in the early 1970's, I knew I had discovered a life-long practice. In many ways it was a "life-saving" practice. From the beginning I connected to a place deep inside; a place I wanted to explore more and more.

Over the years there have been times I could not practice every day. Whenever that occurred, I remembered why Yoga was so important. As a 20-something, I wanted to be fit and able to do all the exotic postures I saw in the Yoga books. There were no teachers near me, and I basically taught myself.

The books I found didn't emphasize the stilling of the mind or the importance of breathing. They offered what might be called today, a Western approach. The physical practice predominated.

Once I had been practicing for a few years, I found a teacher who modeled for me what would become my own teaching style. Her connection with Yoga was like a thread wrapping around me and weaving the ancient wisdom teachings into the fabric of my being.

When I had my children in the 1980's, Yoga helped prepare me for childbirth and offered a few quiet moments in the busy schedule of rearing little ones. My daughter wanted to try Yoga poses from an early age. She loved curling up into Child's Pose while holding her stuffed snow leopard. Bedtime was a special time to lie still and practice breathing.

I remember the first time I practiced Tranquility pose with my son. It was a lazy afternoon and we decided to read a book. I took pillows to the wall and demonstrated how I was going to rest as I read to him. He giggled and sat cross-legged watching me. A few pages into the book, he decided to join me at the wall. This became our favorite pose and it helped us take a break.

One of the most important lessons I learned from my early classes was the idea that any time spent doing Yoga is worth it. Even five minutes would make a difference. In my experience, that is true.

For many years, I practiced every morning for 30-60 minutes. It became such a habit I didn't feel I was ready to leave the house without completing it. During those years, if I was sick or traveling, I might not practice; but I always felt something was missing and returned to the mat as soon as I could.

Yoga is like that. It finds a way into your heart and calls you back again and again. Not simply a physical practice of poses to be performed on a mat, Yoga infuses every aspect of living in day-to-day life. In fact, "practicing Yoga" happens all the time, whether on the mat or not.

It wasn't until the 1990's that I considered becoming a Yoga teacher. My passion and love of Yoga, along with a background in teaching elementary students, combined to nurture what would become the recognition of my deepest heart's desire. Encouraged by my teacher, I enrolled in a two-year home study course, including an intensive training at the Himalayan Institute in Honesdale, Pennsylvania.

I found the more I studied and practiced, the more I wanted to learn. The ancient wisdom teachings are deep and endless. I knew I could study for lifetimes and not absorb it all. Reading about the ancient traditions and the philosophical tenets of Yoga provides a deepening understanding of how Yoga is an intricate part of one's being. For me, the time on the mat and the time off the mat have dissolved into one another. Yoga is a part of each moment. Every class, either as a student or teacher, is another lesson for me. I am honored to share Yoga.

I continue to study with many teachers, including Judith Hanson Lasater, Ph.D., P.T., Richard Miller, Ph.D., Saul David Raye, Rod Stryker, and master teachers at the Himalayan Institute. I am grateful to each for the knowledge and understanding they impart. Along with the poses (asana), breathing (pranayama), and meditation, there are always restful poses that draw me into places of profound peace and stillness.

In 2002, I was fortunate to attend a workshop with Judith and the extensive practice of Restorative Yoga began. She taught how to use various props and how to help students find the position that would bring the most comfort and benefit. Judith offers days of practice with these poses where doing nothing is encouraged. My experience has been that I feel I am being called home each time I practice Restorative Yoga.

Over the years I have found students of all ages and levels of expertise benefit from Restorative Yoga classes. I love teaching these classes and infusing them with meditations, beautiful poetry and ending with a long lavish relaxation. Sharing these practices is the motivation for writing this book.

Life brings a myriad of experiences and lessons. Yoga offers a way to remain centered through emotional storms and physical challenges. Practice that encourages full participation in each moment, Yoga awakens awareness to sensations and feelings perhaps not recognized previously.

For a period of several years I was a caregiver for my mother and my mother-in-law. My schedule was filled with doctor appointments, running errands, and time just visiting. Although it was such a privilege to be present for the end-of-life experience with two women I deeply loved, I often found myself depleted of energy and even anxious or distraught.

Perfect opportunities for Restorative Yoga, I gratefully rolled out my mat to rest in supported poses such as Goddess, Bridge, or Child's Pose. Each posture provides its own nourishment, unique each time you settle into the pose.

Health challenges often appear when we least expect them. A few years ago, I injured myself shoveling snow. This seriously limited my daily Yoga practice. Although I was unable to do even Restorative Yoga, pranayama (breath work) proved to be a lifeline to Yoga.

The breath work brought clarity and contentment to an often frustrating situation. As the swelling in my disc began to recede, I was able to very carefully practice restorative poses such as Supported Shavasana, Supported Half-Dog, Tranquility and a modified Cobra with a support.

I am suggesting through this introduction that Yoga is available to everyone. Restorative Yoga, in particular, can bring you into a new understanding of yourself: your body, mind and spirit. It can be a welcome addition to your daily self-care. I recommend you try a class in your area, if possible. Practice with a qualified teacher is not only enjoyable, but it offers you direction in setting up your props and positioning your body for deep relaxation and optimum benefit.

RESTORATIVE

YOGA

Restful Poses to...

Cradle the Body

Comfort the Heart

Calm the Mind

YOGA

is available

to everyone. Yoga is

the practice of non-striving.

It is accepting yourself, letting go into your

natural flow. The breath is used to help find your

flow and to connect your body, mind and spirit.

Yoga is not about doing, but rather being.

Being in the present moment and

allowing the body/mind to

deeply feel each

sensation.

Chapter 1

Restorative Yoga

Yoga stands apart as a tradition
that has always recognized the importance of the body
and mind living in harmonious relationship to each other.
~Donna Farhi

What is Yoga?

Yoga is generally described as an ancient, holistic approach to health and well-being. Its roots are found in India where it has been practiced for thousands of years. Originally, Yoga evolved as a way to refine the body/mind in preparation for meditation. Today there are almost as many definitions as there are teachers of Yoga. In the West, Yoga is often thought of as a series of physical postures and stretching exercises. Of course, this is only a small fraction of what Yoga is.

One of Yoga's most revered texts, the Yoga Sutra of Patanjali, defines Yoga as "the stilling of the fluctuations of the mind." It is a state of calmness and connection with our true nature, our inner light of awareness. It offers a time-tested path to knowing who we are and living each moment as a new discovery. Truly, Yoga is a way of life.

According to Nicholai Bachman, author of *The Yoga Sutras, An Essential Guide to the Heart of Yoga Philosophy,* Yoga is a set of tools for refining and stabilizing the body, breath, mind and heart. These tools enable you to turn inward to discover your own true nature. Yoga is also characterized as the state of mind in which thoughts and emotions do not distract one's attention. This stillness of the mind allows the inner radiance inherent in each of us to shine.

Judith Hanson Lasater, Ph.D., P.T., author of *Relax and Renew: Restful Yoga for Stressful Times,* defines Yoga as "fundamentally an act of kindness toward oneself." (Notes from workshop, Lisle, IL: 2013)

Typically taught or practiced as a series of poses coordinating the breath and actively moving the body, Yoga sessions end with relaxation. Most often the final pose is Shavasana, or corpse pose. It is the quintessential asana (pose) to experience the essence of Yoga. During Shavasana there is time to receive and to integrate all of the movements and energy of the practice. In Restorative Yoga, each posture throughout the entire practice encourages relaxation.

What is Restorative Yoga?

Restorative Yoga was popularized by Judith Hanson Lasater, Ph.D., P.T., and is based on postures she learned from her teacher, B.K.S. Iyengar. One of the most influential Yoga masters, Iyengar taught in the West for over 60 years. He encouraged his students to use props to avoid strain or injury. This inspired Lasater to formalize a restorative practice.

These restorative poses support your body and bring it into balance by both stimulating and relaxing it. The effects of these soothing, calming poses allow the body to find its innate internal healing process. Some postures may target a particular area such as the hips or the heart, while others are beneficial in a more holistic sense. All create specific responses that can reduce the effects of stress and bring greater health and well-being.

Generally, restorative poses are for times when you feel fatigued or stressed. You can practice when you are ill, or recovering from illness or injury. These poses can be especially helpful during or after major life events, such as the death of a loved one, a change of job or career, marriage or divorce. Major holidays, family events and even vacations can be stressful. These postures can be used to nurture and comfort you in any circumstance life may bring to you.

Yoga, in whatever form, has a profound effect on your nervous system. The Autonomic Nervous System (ANS) consists of the Sympathetic Nervous System (SNS) and the Parasympathetic Nervous System (PNS). SNS prepares your body for action. PNS calms your nerves and brings a return to balance. Together the whole ANS regulates several body processes that are usually below the level of consciousness. One of these processes, breathing, operates both consciously and unconsciously.

During the practice of Yoga, the combination of the pose and the breath triggers the PNS. This can reduce your heart rate, lower blood pressure and quiet the mind. It also stimulates your immune system and contributes to the optimum function of your endocrine system. Your body/mind comes into balance.

What does Restorative Yoga do?

1) Uses a variety of props to support deep relaxation.
2) Encourages the spine to stretch gently in all

directions: backbends, forward bends, twists, laterals and inverted poses.

3) Stimulates and soothes the internal organs. For instance, a forward bend squeezes the belly, forcing the blood out, and when released allows fresh oxygenated blood to flow into the area.

4) Opens the front side of the body giving space to the body.

5) Reverses the effects of gravity giving the heart a rest and drawing blood and lymphatic fluids from the lower body into the upper body. Inversions restore tired legs and feet, soothe the nerves and reduce the systemic effects of stress.

6) Balances two aspects of Prana, or life force, that are carried on the breath. When balanced, the result is a calm and energized body/mind.

Why Restorative Yoga?

In our busy, often hectic lifestyles, we have forgotten how to relax, to rest deeply. Even in deep sleep, tension is still experienced. But in the state of true relaxation, there is no movement, the brain is quiet and there is a dynamic calm. Here is the best part: relaxation is something you can learn, and it is the healthiest thing you can do for yourself.

Your mind is always busy thinking; it's what the mind does. The ancient teachings of Yoga tell us you are not your mind; rather your mind is an instrument for you to experience life. As long as you remain identified with your thoughts, they will bring stress and suffering. Learning to relax allows you to observe the body/mind and recognize you are not your thoughts or your body, but something deeper.

From the nondual perspective, Yoga is a practice of letting go and being the pure Presence that you are. Richard Miller, Ph.D., author of *Yoga Nidra, the Meditative Heart of Yoga*, writes there is a stillness out of which everything arises and returns. We are this stillness. Too often we are so attached to all of the objects arising out of the stillness that we have forgotten who we are.

The approach to the restorative series presented in this book is the practice of letting go and simply being in the present moment. There are three points of emphasis: the pose, the breath, and the feeling mind, all coalescing into Presence. It is the practice of not doing, just being.

You use a variety of props and position your body so with minimal effort, you receive the benefits. The idea is to rest in the pose allowing gravity and the props to draw your body into the deep stretches and openings associated with each pose. In this way you are able to welcome all the sensations in the body while resting and nourishing the body/mind at a very deep level. All of the body's systems benefit from this deep relaxation.

Supported poses tone the body with minimum effort and have a powerful effect. They nourish the glands of the endocrine system, soothe the nervous system, and allow the inner organs space to be gently massaged. The benefits of these postures are essential for total health and well-being.

Restorative Yoga

is the practice of finding your way to

rest and relaxation.

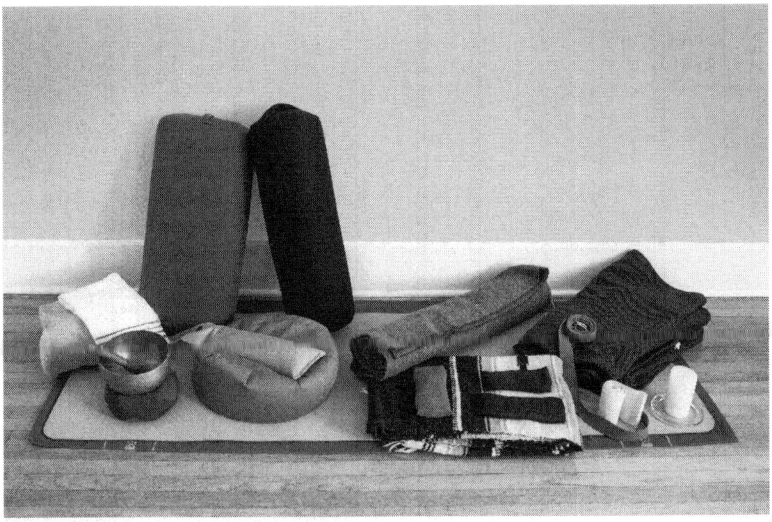

Commonly used Yoga props

Chapter 2

Prepare for Practice

Settle in the here and now.
reach down into the center
where the world is not spinning
and drink this holy peace.
~Danna Faulds

Begin by gathering the props necessary to be as comfortable as possible: a mat, blankets, bolsters, zafu (round meditation cushion), eye bag, and perhaps pillows, towels, and a strap. Props offer unique ways to assist you to find "deliberate stillness" in each pose. (*Relax and Renew,* p. 23)

Blankets are such versatile props and may be folded in any number of ways. For Restorative Yoga firm, tightly-woven wool or cotton blankets are best. Fluffy comforters or afghans will not hold the desired shape or be firm enough to be supportive.

Each blanket can be folded lengthwise, and then folded back and forth accordion style to end with a stacked blanket measuring approximately 30x12x6 inches. It can be used to support the spine, knees or head. The folded blanket fits the width of the mat and supports the body. Blankets may be stacked to create higher props.

Two or three folded blankets are usually equivalent to the height of a standard rectangular bolster.

You can roll the blanket to support the neck or to use under the knees. It does not need to be completely rolled if the finished shape is too thick for your body to be comfortable.

For example, when first practicing a simple backbend, Supported Fish, you may feel an arch in the upper back with one or two rolls of the blanket. As the chest opens and the upper back becomes more flexible, you may decide to roll the blanket several times. Eventually you may wish to replace the rolled blanket with a bolster for an even deeper opening of the heart center.

The Appendix contains a chart illustrating the most common ways the blankets are used. As not everyone has the Yoga props described in this book, options are listed on the chart as well. (p. 139)

Other props include a non-skid mat (usually 68x24 inches), a zafu or firm round cushion, a bolster (rectangular or round), and an eye bag. Eye bags are commonly silk or cotton and filled with uncooked rice, flaxseeds, or hypoallergenic plastic beads. Many include soothing herbs such as lavender or chamomile.

Extra pillows (square, round or oblong in shape) are useful for several poses. Towels can also be used to support ankles, knees, arms, head or neck.

Once your props are ready, find a quiet place to practice. Unroll your mat, come to the floor and move into a restful position on your back. Place a rolled blanket, bolster or zafu under your knees to support your lower back. If necessary, support the neck with a small pillow or rolled towel. Make certain your body is at ease and comfortable and your breathing is natural. Finally, place a soft eye bag over the eyes to relax not only the eyes, but the forehead and all the muscles around the eyes.

Next, take time for body and breath awareness. These two techniques are crucial to your practice. Even if you have time for only one pose, you need to prepare the body/mind.

Body Awareness

Beginning with a deep awareness of the body/mind, welcome sounds, smells, colors, light and the touch of air on the skin. Turn inward and notice sensations inside the body and mind. Scan the body beginning with the jaw. Notice sensations in the jaw, mouth, ears, nose, and eyes. Move attention to the forehead, scalp, back of the head, and back of the neck. Take time to sense the inner walls of the throat and the tongue.

Notice the right shoulder, upper arm, elbow, lower arm, wrist, hand, thumb, index finger, middle finger, ring finger, little finger, palm of the right hand, back of the hand, and the entire hand.

Bring awareness to the left shoulder, upper arm, elbow, lower arm, wrist, hand, thumb, index finger, middle finger, ring finger, little finger, palm of the left hand, back of the hand, and the entire hand. Feel both arms and palms.

Move into the torso and notice the chest, the heart, lungs, ribcage, the upper back and along the spine. Bring attention into the solar plexus, the space just above the naval and notice the internal organs, the space inside the body.

Then move awareness to the area below the naval and sense whatever sensations are present in the pelvis, the sacrum and backside of the body. Move into the right hip socket. Feel the space in this joint. Sense the upper leg, the hamstrings and the quadriceps. Become aware of the knee, front and back, the lower leg, ankle, right foot, big toe, second toe, third toe, fourth toe, and little toe.

Now become aware of the left hip. Feel the space in this joint. Move into the upper leg, noticing the hamstrings and the quadriceps. Become aware of the knee, front and back, the lower leg, ankle, left foot, big toe, second toe, third toe, fourth toe, and little toe.

Notice the entire body, feel vibrant sensations shimmering everywhere.

Did you know
there are areas in our bodies with
concentrated nerve fibers? The yogis discovered
thousands of years ago when we systematically bring
awareness to particular areas of the body,
we can awaken sensation and let go
of tension at the same time.

Body awareness
enhances our ability to be both
alert and relaxed.

Body awareness
awakens us to the experience
that we are more than a physical body.
We are radiant vibration ~
an energy field.

Breath Awareness

In Yoga, the breath always leads the way. Begin by becoming aware of your breath flowing through the nostrils at a slow even rate. As you bring attention to the breath, it will automatically begin to deepen and lengthen. The breath must never be forced. Find the flow that is natural, comfortable and effortless. Stay with this awareness of the breath throughout the practice. Each moment, bring awareness back to the breath. Follow the breath into the present moment. This is where all of the healing, nourishing, restoring and energizing takes place.

If your mind wants to wander, and it usually does, simply bring it back to the breath each time it strays. Staying with the breath is one of the most important elements of a restorative practice.

If you do nothing but lie on your back and breathe, you will derive untold benefits. Even so, the human body needs to be used and moving the body in these postures will bring harmony and balance to body, mind and spirit.

"The human body is a complex spiritual instrument. Ordinary physical breathing is not only the exchange of oxygen and carbon dioxide; it is the link to our light body. With every inhale-exhale a parallel energy flow in our light body is occurring. Bringing attention to the outer breath cultivates a growing awareness of this inner breath, harmonizes these interpenetrating bodies and quiets the mind. In breath the visible and the invisible worlds meet."

The Illuminated Prayer, Coleman Barks and Michael Green

Tune in to the sensations in the body/mind. Let awareness scan your body for places that are open and relaxed and those that are tense or tight and closed. Feel the breath flow over and through the body like a wave. And let the breath move the body into each pose. Continue to return to the breath. Move from deep inside. Let each pose unfold.

Watching the breath

is the way to focus on the present

moment. Begin by inhaling through the

nostrils and feeling the sensation of air inside the body.

Let the belly fill with breath. Notice all of the

sensations. Move deep inside and feel each sensation.

Your body will know when to exhale. Follow

the flow of breath all the way out

of your body. Feel how

empty the space

inside your

body

is.

Chapter 3

Strengthen Your Spine

To truly relax is to simply be...
These poses support and bring balance, allowing the body/mind to move into its natural healing process.
~Nancy Hodge Long

The basic restorative series presented here includes a combination of seven postures designed to move the spine in all directions. Beginning in a resting pose, you move from one gentle backbend, *Supported Fish Pose*, to another *Supported Goddess Pose. Supported Crescent Moon Pose* provides a lateral side stretch followed by *Reclining Twist with a Bolster Pose*, a gentle twist. Then let the body rest deeply in a forward bend, *Supported Child's Pose. Tranquility Pose* offers a gentle inversion to reverse the effects of gravity on the body bringing calm and serenity. Return to your resting position, *Supported Shavasana Pose*, to complete the practice.

Begin with body and breath awareness as described in the previous chapter. Focus your attention on all of the sensations present in the body. This deep connection to the body promotes relaxation by connecting with specific places in the body where there may be tension, tightness or other sensations. One of the simplest ways to become aware of the body is through the breath. Use the breath to notice the body, then let the body dissolve into your breath.

Of the many breathing techniques available, the one described in Chapter 2 combines body awareness to bring a deep connection to the present moment. One aspect of breath awareness facilitates the surrender of the body/mind, allowing whatever is present to arise and dissolve without trying to control or manipulate the breath.

To let go of tension,

especially in the back body is a gift.

We all hold tension

and to be able to release the tight muscles

along the spine is sweet indeed.

Bringing the breath

into these areas

allows healing energy

to penetrate the body at a cellular level

renewing body, mind and spirit.

(1) Supported Fish Pose

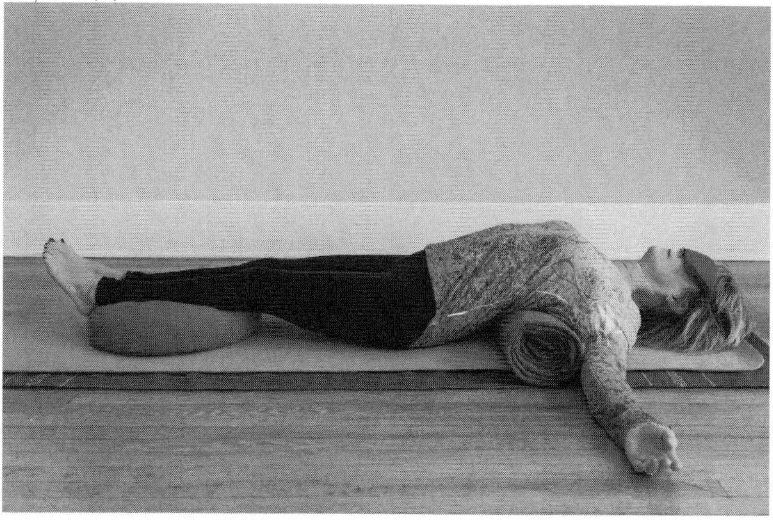

Props:

Rolled blanket or bolster
Zafu or rolled blanket
Rolled towel or small neck pillow
Eye bag

Time:

1-3 minutes, building to 5-7

Benefits:

Counter pose for rounded spine
Energizes the front body
Stimulates the internal organs
Lengthens the spine
Deep muscular stretch of the back

Cautions: Do not practice if ~

Your back has pain as you lie in the pose
You have diagnosed disc disease

You are more than 3 months pregnant

This gentle backbend gives your body welcome relief from the normal way the body is held with rounded shoulders and collapsed chest. We sit and stand with a rounded spine for so many activities (driving, working at the computer or preparing a meal in the kitchen), muscle tension accumulates in the shoulders and upper back. This pose is a very useful counter movement.

To prepare for this pose gather the necessary props: a bolster or rolled blanket, a cushion, and an eye bag. The bolster or rolled blanket will be directly under the shoulder blades. To come into this position in a safe way, lie down on one side of your body and roll onto the bolster or blanket. If the upper back is uncomfortable or it is difficult to breathe, the bolster or rolled blanket is too thick. The rolled blanket can be adjusted by unrolling it until a comfortable arch is formed in the upper back. If a deeper backbend is appropriate, switch to a bolster. Adjust your body so a slight arch in the upper back is felt and the breath remains smooth and easy. Place another cushion or zafu under the knees to relieve any discomfort in your lower back.

Check to see that the cervical spine is comfortable. If there is any discomfort or if your chin is drawing upward toward the ceiling, add a small pillow or neck roll (a rolled towel works nicely) to maintain the natural curve of the neck.

Bring your arms out to rest on the floor at the "T" position, above the support. Stay still for a few breaths to make certain your body is comfortable. If there is any discomfort, please move off of the support and make whatever adjustment necessary to relieve the strain. Once the position is found, place the eye bag over the eyes and allow your body to sink into the floor and the supports.

Notice the breath. As the mind rests in the breath, the body softens. Become aware of places that may be tense or tight and places where the breath flows easily. Once the breath has found a slow, even rhythm, begin a systematic progression through the body to consciously let go of any tension or discomfort.

Swallow and release any constriction in the throat. Allow your jaw to soften and feel the tongue floating in the mouth. Notice the sensations, the energy in the mouth and the pool of sensation in the hollow at the center of the tongue. Feel the skin of your face soften and let the eyes rest back deep in the hollows of their sockets. Release any tension in the eyebrows and feel all the muscles around the eyes soften. Let the forehead feel like a wide ribbon of satin and allow your brain to "float" inside the skull. Resting on the center of the back of the head, feel your whole face and head melting into the support beneath.

Now bring attention to your hands noticing feelings of warmth or coolness, tingling or movement. Let them rest, fingers barely curling. Feel a pool of sensation in the palm of each hand radiating out through the fingers. As awareness moves up the arms notice the sensation of heaviness. Let the arms be heavy and the muscles just drop away from the bones.

Notice your arms reaching out from the center of your chest. With each inhalation, the front body opens; with the exhale, the belly and internal organs soften and the mind quiets. Allow the back to sink deeper into the props. As your back body releases, feel the pelvis soften and the hip sockets become spacious. The legs become heavy and the feet flop open about hip-width apart.

Consider a place where you feel safe and at ease. Go to that place as you lie in this pose. Allow the body/mind to be nourished and comforted. Begin by practicing for 1-3 minutes. As you become familiar with the pose, you may wish to remain in it for 5-7 minutes.

Gradually bring awareness into the body. Begin to move slowly, rolling onto the right side and resting briefly before coming up to a seated position.

This pose is an antidote for rounding the spine. It energizes the front body, stimulates the internal organs and lengthens the spine allowing for a deep muscular stretch of the back. Refreshed and energized, move on to the next pose.

(2) Supported Goddess Pose

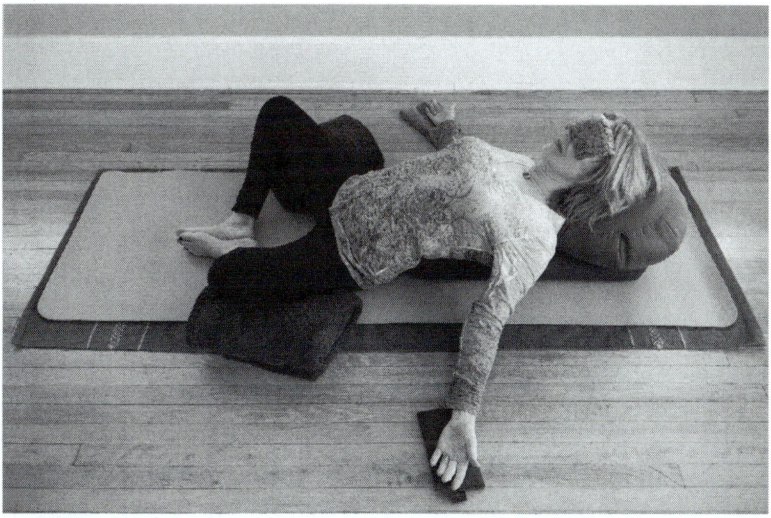

Props:

- Bolster
- Zafu
- 2 blankets or soft pillows
- eye bag
- belt or strap
- 2 extra pillows

Time:

- 7-10 minutes

Benefits:

- Helps balance blood pressure
- Improves circulation and respiration
- Relieves headaches
- Frees abdominal and pelvic restrictions

Cautions:

- If you feel stiff after this pose, practice for less time.

Thighs must be supported if you have knee problems.

Supported Goddess (Bound-Angle or *Cobbler) Pose* is considered one of the most important in the series. Physically, it opens the entire front body - chest, belly and pelvis. These are areas that are often restricted by the ways we sit and stand and even the way our clothes fit. On a mental-emotional level, this pose allows for a deep opening with safety and security. The whole body is cradled by the props as the chest and front torso gently open, allowing for an opening inside the body as well.

Judith Hanson Lasater, Ph.D., P.T., refers to Patanjali's Yoga Sutra and the description of hiranyagarbha, the Sanskrit word meaning "the great golden womb of the universe." The entire universe is held within this golden womb. Lasater writes, "As we practice Supported Bound-Angle Pose, we are reminded of this primordial place of complete rest and ultimate protection." The experience of being held by this force is "profoundly comforting" and brings a deep sense of "equanimity and well-being." (*Relax and Renew,* pp. 33-34)

Preparing for this pose takes time, patience and a lot of props. Do not be discouraged. The results of this pose will not be a disappointment. Assemble the necessary props and sit in front of the short end of the bolster with the tailbone touching it. Bring the soles of your feet together with knees bent in cobbler pose. (See photo p. 19)

Place a pillow or rolled blanket under each thigh so the legs and hips are totally supported. Even if you are supple and can open easily in *Cobbler Pose,* you need to support the weight of your legs. Care must be taken to avoid injuring or even straining the ligaments connecting the hips to the spine. The objective is to open the chest and relax the belly, rather than overstretch the inner thighs.

Use your arms for support as you lower the torso onto the bolster. Place a zafu under your head to support your head and neck. Make certain that your spine is comfortable and you are supporting the sacrum. You may need another zafu or a pillow to support the spine.

Pillows or folded blankets may be placed under each arm to enhance the feeling of letting go. This will relieve any tension in the neck and arms and relax the shoulders. Make sure the head and neck are supported. The forehead should be higher than the breastbone, and breastbone higher than pubic bone. The final position has your torso at a 45-degree angle to the floor.

As a variation to prevent the feet from sliding away from the body, you may use a strap. (See p. 97) Fasten the strap into a loop large enough to fit around the hips and feet. Take the strap over your head and adjust it around the hips; then wrap the strap around the feet, soles touching. This should simply hold the feet in place and allow them to relax without sliding away. Place an eye bag over your eyes and prepare to move into a deep state of relaxation.

Bring awareness into the breath and feel the flow of the breath as it enters the nostrils and moves deep into the chest, expanding into the belly. As you exhale, feel the whole body soften. Focus your awareness inside the body and feel the inner space grow with each breath. Rest into the vast spaciousness inside the body. Let the body/mind float on the breath as it moves in and out slowly, smoothly and evenly.

Consider being held in the great golden womb of the Universe. Remain in the pose for 7-10 minutes. After relaxing so deeply, allow the body/mind to return slowly. Move deliberately in order to have the deep sense of peace fill every fiber of your being.

Supported Goddess Pose is helpful for those with high blood pressure, headaches, or breathing problems. It improves respiration and circulation. Areas of constriction and tension in the pelvis and abdomen are freed, allowing space for the internal organs to relax.

(3) Supported Crescent Moon Pose

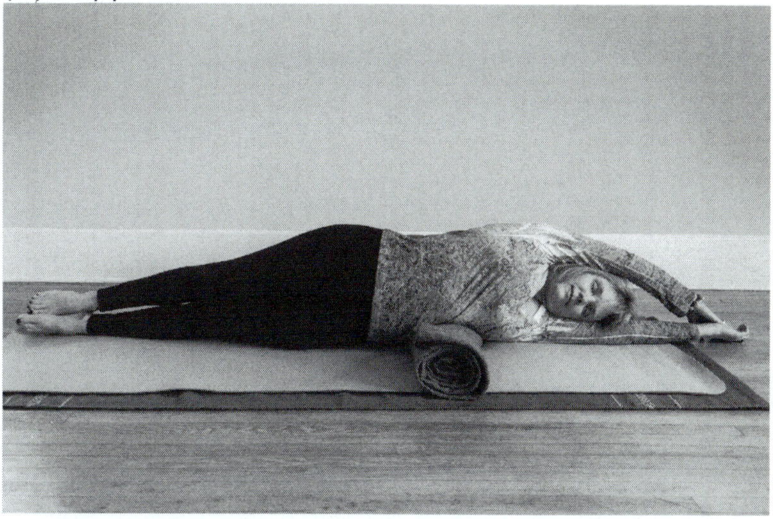

Props:

Bolster or rolled blanket
Eye bag
Small rolled towel, if needed

Time:

1-2 minutes on each side

Benefits:

Stretches the side body
Stimulates internal organs
Improves respiration
Relieves stress and anxiety

Cautions:

Be careful not to overstretch
Make sure you are supporting your neck

In this pose, the spine is extended laterally, bringing a welcome stretch to the side body. A rolled blanket or a bolster is placed horizontally at the edge of the right hip. With knees bent, slowly come to rest on the prop with the floating ribs on the right side of the body centered on the prop. With the right arm outstretched, palm upward on the floor, rest the side of head on the upper arm. Bring the left arm overhead and let the palms come together in prayer position. Feel the entire left side of the body stretch and open. Remember to move into the pose in a very slow and deliberate way. As you settle onto the props, allow the body to open slowly.

If the neck is uncomfortable, place a small rolled towel or pillow between it and your arm. If the stretch is too much, adjust the bolster or exchange it for a rolled blanket. Always tune into how the body feels before continuing. Complete the pose by straightening the legs for a deeper stretch. Enjoy the stretch in the entire left side of the body. Relax into the posture as the breath becomes more effortless.

Allow the breath to move into the torso and expand the left side body. With each breath, notice the opening between the ribs increase and allow any places of tension or tightness to be dissolved. After 1-2 minutes, release the arms and slowly move to the other side. Breathe into the stretch and feel the right side of the body open.

Lateral poses give attention to an overlooked part of the torso. They stimulate the internal organs, elongate the side body, and bring oxygen into this part of the body. They help relieve stress and anxiety as the torso opens.

(4) Reclining Twist with Bolster Pose

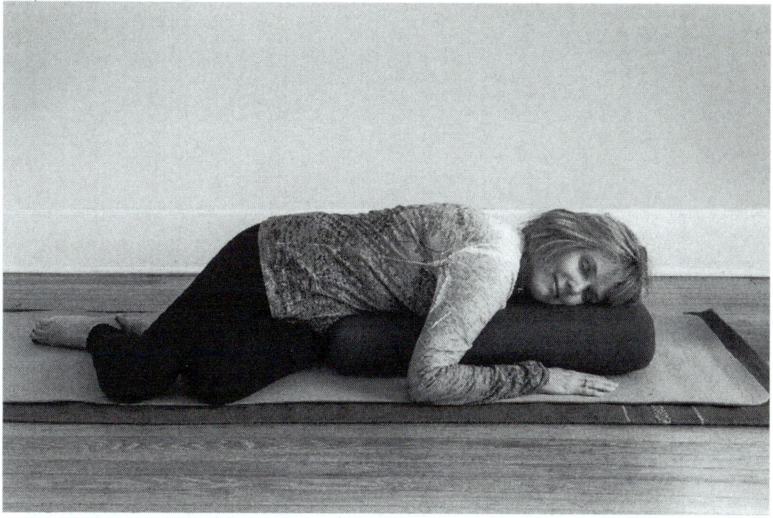

Props:

Bolster
Eye bag
Blanket or pillow

Time:

2 minutes on each side

Benefits:

Relieves tightness in the back muscles
Encourages a gentle spiraling of the spine
Cleanses and refreshes organs and glands
Maintains the health of spinal discs and joints

Cautions:

Proceed with caution if you have any back injury, disc disease or chronic sacroiliac problems

Twisting poses release tension and blocks along the spine, providing a deep release as the entire spine spirals. This allows the muscles of the back and the sides of the body to soften and gently stretch. The intercostal muscles stretch to bring space between the ribs and open the body for enhanced breathing.

This supported variation brings an opportunity to untie all of the knots in the body/mind. Gently twisting the body allows the mind to unwind, emotional knots in the body can untangle and the natural flow of energy returns.

Begin sitting with a rectangular bolster (or a stack of 2-3 blankets) placed at the edge of the right hip, knees bent, feet move to the left so the legs rest on each other. As the body slowly makes its way to the bolster, feel the body lengthen and twist to the right. Let the hands find the floor on either side of the bolster. With the elbows bending, slowly lower your chest onto the bolster as the arms find a comfortable position to rest.

Notice the upper back turning toward the right as the knees point to the left, bringing a slight spiral into the spine. The head may be placed with either cheek resting on the support. If there is any discomfort in the neck, place an additional pillow, zafu, or rolled towel to support the head. When the head is turned to the right, the twist is deeper.

Rest on the bolster. Find the breath and begin to follow the flow of the inhalation and exhalation. Let the breath move into the upper back, noticing places that may be tense or tight. Soften the space between the shoulder blades. With the inhale, feel the inner space expand and soften. Each exhale reminds the body to release into the twist. Allow the body to become longer and longer as gravity draws it deeply into the support. Let the breath be natural and effortless.

This pose needs only a brief time (1-2 minutes) on each side to be effective. Move out of the pose carefully by first turning your head to the left for a breath or two. Place the palms on the floor and gently press down to lift off of the bolster. Allow the body to sit briefly before moving to the other side. When the pose is completed on the second side, rest for a breath or two before returning to a seated position.

Twists benefit the circulatory system and internal organs as well as the musculoskeletal system. They have a cleansing and refreshing effect on internal organs and glands. Additionally, twists help maintain the health of discs and joints on the back of the spine.

So often

the mind twists itself into such knots

we hardly recognize ourselves or anything else.

Twisting the body

gives us the chance to let go of

all the mental

and emotional knots.

Then the natural healing process begins.

(5) Supported Child's Pose

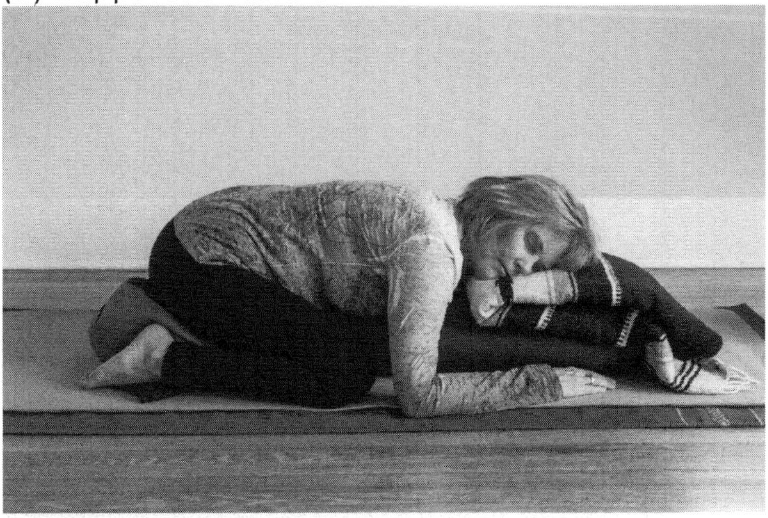

Props:

Bolster or stack of 2-3 blankets
Zafu or long-roll blanket

Time:

3-4 minutes with head to each cheek

Benefits:

Improves breathing by opening the back
Eases tension in the back
Releases the hip and shoulder joints
Soothes the nervous system
Quiets the mind

Cautions:

Protect knees, ankles and feet
Limit practice if you have a severe back condition
Do not do this pose if more than 3 months pregnant

From a seated position, come onto all fours. Feel the flow of the breath moving through the body. Stay with the feelings and sensations in the body/mind. Relax the hips back toward the heels and separate the knees, allow the big toes to move toward one another and possibly touch. Slide a bolster or stack of 2-3 blankets vertically between the legs and let the torso soften onto the prop. Support the head with 1-2 folded blankets or towels so that the head rests comfortably on the right cheek. (Halfway through the pose turn and rest on the left cheek.)

Allow the body to find a position where your arms are resting comfortably. Slip a pillow or zafu in the space between the buttocks and the heels. Lift your hips slightly to allow the placement of the cushion and then feel the pelvis melt into the support.

Once the props are in place use the breath to determine whether any adjustments are necessary. If there is any tension or discomfort, take time to move, remove, or add supports. Settle into the pose as the body/mind softens into the supports.

With each breath, encourage every cell in your body to soften and unclench. Invite gravity to draw the legs down into the earth as the thighs, hips, and pelvis become spacious and open. Soften the low back and feel the tailbone move toward the heels. Simultaneously, feel the shoulder blades widen like wings and the whole upper back open into the vast spaciousness inside the body. Feel the arms dangling from the shoulder joints that have softened and expanded.

Allow the body/mind to soften and unwind. Rest the eyes into the hollows of the eye sockets, release the jaw, soften the tongue and unfurl the brow. Dissolve the armor around your back so that the skin feels soft and smooth, like a satin comforter covering you. Encourage the entire body to feel spacious, open and at ease.

The torso may relax enough to lengthen the spine more. Let your hands press into the floor lifting the torso just enough to slide the belly toward the heart, the heart toward the head, and the top of the head toward the edge of the support. Lengthen your spine as the torso returns to rest on the props.

This pose provides the chance to use the breath to move even deeper into the body's vast, tranquil inner space. Feel the sensations of breath expanding into your back. The shoulder blades and back of the waist rise spreading with the inhalation and melting toward the support on the exhalation. The inhalations are long and wide filling all the spaces of the back, while exhalations are warm and endless. Simply enjoy the serenity and easy rhythm of the breath flowing in and out of the body.

After 3-4 minutes (halfway through the pose), turn your head and rest on the opposite cheek. Let the support cradle the head so the shoulders can release. Feel the heart melting into the bolster and soften the belly. Allow the world to dissolve as awareness draws inward toward the center of being. With every muscle, bone, organ, tissue and cell softening, surrender to that deep ocean of tranquility.

Child's Pose is one of Yoga's classic resting postures. It improves breathing by bringing awareness of the breath into the back of the body. It eases tension in the back and releases the hip joints. The mind is quieted, while the nervous system is soothed. There is a sense of feeling safe and protected, offering shelter from the troubles of the world.

(6) Supported Tranquility Pose

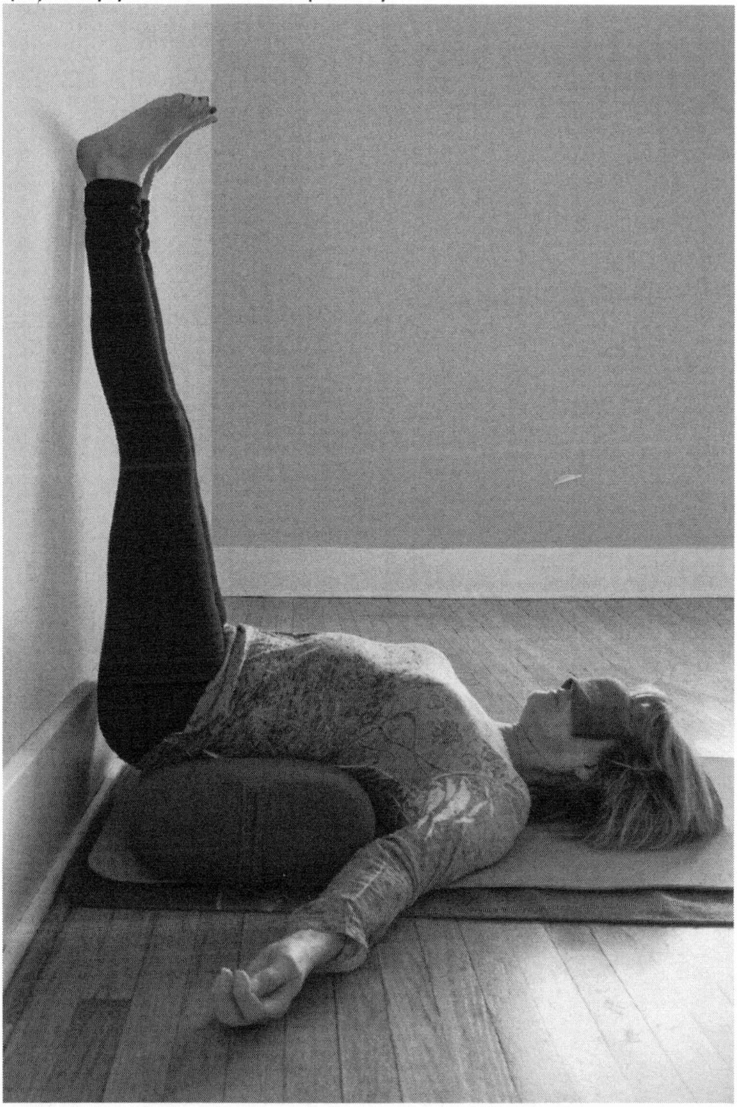

Props:

- Bolster or zafu
- 1 or more folded blankets or towels
- Eye bag

Time:

5-10 minutes

Benefits:

Restores tired legs and feet
Soothes the nervous system
Quiets the mind
Relieves headaches
Balances blood pressure
Regulates the thyroid gland

Cautions:

Not recommended for those who should avoid inversions, if you have hiatal hernia, eye pressure, retinal problems, heart condition, neck injury or are menstruating.

If this pose creates pressure in the head, do not do it.

If discomfort in the back, bend the knees and place your feet on a wall or loosely cross your ankles and let the wall support you.

Supported Tranquility Pose is a gentle inversion in which the pelvis and torso rest in a slight backbend and the legs hang above the heart. Legs may rest against a wall or just extend into the air above the hips. (See p. 99) As in all inversions, gravity plays a central part in reversing the usual position of the body in space. Inversions are beneficial and essential to a complete practice. Those with contraindications, may wish to substitute *Supported Shavasana with Legs on a Chair.* (See p. 52)

To prepare for this pose, sit with the right side of the body against the wall and place a support next to the left hip. Come onto the floor and swing the legs up onto the wall. The sitting bones should be as close to the wall as comfortable. The tighter the hamstrings, the more space may be needed between the wall and the body.

Once the legs are on the wall, bend the knees and press the soles of the feet into the wall to elevate the hips. Slide the cushion under and rest back on the support. Make whatever adjustments necessary to be comfortable.

If it is difficult to maintain this position, try the pose against the wall. With the wall supporting the legs, any need for holding them in the air is gone.

For this variation, lie on your back with knees bent and feet close to the hips. Press your feet into the floor allowing the hips to lift, slide a zafu or bolster under the hips and let them sink into the support. If there is any discomfort, place the feet back on the floor and lift the hips. Rearrange the support until the buttocks, hips and pelvis are completely at ease.

Slowly feel the legs reach upward until they are hanging in the air above the hips. It is important they are directly above the hips in order for gravity to draw the top of the leg into the hip socket. The perfect placement is found when your legs rest in the air with little muscular contraction. The weight of the legs release both the hip joints and the lower back.

It is important that your neck is positioned to preserve its natural curve. If there is any strain or if the chin feels it is pressing into your chest, use a small rolled towel or neck pillow to support it. The prop should support the vertebra (C7) at the base of the neck near the shoulders, and not be placed in the center of the neck where the curve is the greatest.

Once your body has settled into the posture, bring awareness into the breath. Let the breath flow to the tips of the toes and back to the crown of the head. Forget the external world for the next several minutes and do nothing. Doing nothing is a most important task for restoring balance and well-being to the body, mind and spirit.

Scan your body for any residue of tension. Feel it dissolve into the lovely pool created by the legs draining into the belly. Let the brain become tranquil, releasing any worries or fears that may be lingering. Notice the breath. Inhale, observing the belly fill and exhale, all the fatigue washing out of the body. Let your body ride the waves of the breath inviting the breath to deepen even more.

Become aware of the slight pause at the end of the exhalation and again at the end of the inhalation. In this brief moment of stillness, feel the tranquility and deep rest of utter silence. Each breath brings a stillness, a moment of just being.

You may practice this posture for 7-10 minutes. When ready, begin the process of returning to an upright position with deliberate attention. If your legs are hanging in the air without support of a wall, bring the feet to your mat, hip distance apart. If you are at the wall, place your feet on it with your knees bent. Press the feet into the floor or the wall, as appropriate, and lift the hips just enough to remove the support. Slowly bring the hips back to the floor and roll to one side keeping the body curled in a fetal position. Take a breath or two before coming to a seated position. Remember to use your arms to lift the torso so that you do not strain your lower back.

7) Supported Shavasana Pose

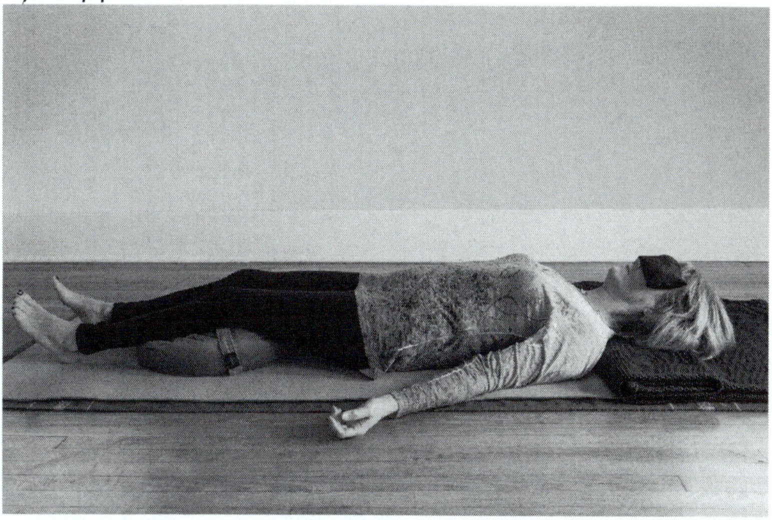

Props:

- Blanket
- Zafu or bolster
- Eye bag

Time:

- 5-10 minutes

Benefits:

- Relieves tension in lower back and abdomen
- Brings a sense of well-being and wholeness

Cautions:

- If more than 3 months pregnant, lie on your side.

Supported Shavasana Pose, the final posture in this series, is also called corpse pose. It offers you the chance to lie still and withdraw your attention from the objects of the five senses. The pose mimics a corpse, encouraging your body to be still. Resting on the back, you become aware of body sensations and thoughts floating through the mind. Be detached from these thoughts and simply watch.

The ultimate posture for relaxing body, mind, and spirit, *Shavasana* can bring a deep sense of calm and connection to those who practice it consistently. It is considered by many Yoga teachers to be the quintessential pose. It is the very best one to help reduce stress, tension, anxiety, and fatigue. In fact, if you have time for only one pose, this is the one to choose.

In this restorative practice, use whatever props you need for complete comfort. This may include a bolster or zafu under the knees to release pressure on the lower back, and perhaps a rolled towel under the neck or a small pillow under the head to maintain the natural curve of the neck. Although it is important the spine is aligned with the head and hips, the body's comfort is of primary consideration.

Begin by finding the breath and allowing it to move slowly through the body. Come into a deep sense of its rhythm. Fill and expand the body as you inhale and soften. Let go of all tension or discomfort on the exhale. Once your body has found equanimity, tune into the sensations that arise. Notice the mouth and all the sensations inside the mouth, the teeth, tongue, jaw and gums. Let your tongue relax; feel it all the way into the root of the tongue.

Soften the skin of the face and let your head rest back into the prop or floor beneath it. Feel the forehead soften and notice the space inside the skull. It may feel as if the brain is floating.

Feel sensations in the ears. Let the ears become funnels of vibrant energy and be aware of the folds and valleys of the external ears. Notice the eyes and consciously allow them to rest deeply into the sockets. Feel the muscles all around your eyes soften.

Let the radiance of the eyes flow in a stream of energy through the back of the head and down the neck until the sensations of the throat can be identified. Swallow and release any tightness and let this whole area soften.

Move into the palms of both hands and allow the sensations to form a pool of energy in the center of each. Notice how energy radiates from these pools into all the fingers, moving out through the tips. Feel the energy body surrounding your physical body and gently vibrating into all the cells, tissues, organs, bones and muscles.

Feel the torso and the center of the chest. Let the energetic sensations fill the heart and radiate through the entire torso. Continue moving through the body: into the belly; the backside of the body; the hips and pelvis; and into the legs, ankles, and feet. Feel your whole body soften and let go into this vast inner spaciousness.

Remain in this pose for at least five minutes, and longer if possible. Of all Yoga poses, this is the premier posture for bringing wholeness and radiant health to body, mind and spirit.

When ready, let the body/mind return to a conscious state. Move slowly and deliberately as you come to a seated position. Take a few minutes to notice how you feel and then remember why you are practicing Restorative Yoga. Find just one thing that you are grateful for in this moment and let it rest in your heart.

Ahh ~

Shavasana brings absolute rest.

It is a symbolic dying to all distractions ~

inner and outer. It offers stillness.

And in stillness resides

All That Is.

Chapter 4

Pamper Your Back

Not going, not coming
rooted, deep and still
not reaching out, not reaching in
just resting, at the center...
~Shih-Te

This series focuses on ways to release tension in the lower spine, to let go of anxiety and worry, and to bring spaciousness to the lower half of the body.

The five poses are systematically designed to stretch, release and comfort the low back. First, *Supported Half-Dog Pose* relaxes the legs, abdomen, and lower back, while releasing tension in the upper back. *Supported Fish Pose* opens your chest and releases tension along the entire spine. Next, *Elevated Twist Pose* offers relief to the small muscles and ligaments of the lower back. *Supported Child's Pose* is an excellent way to stretch the long muscles of the lower back and pelvis, while relaxing the abdomen. The ending pose, *Shavasana with Legs on a Chair*, removes pressure from the lower back and allows the body to come into a safe, nurturing position.

Before beginning this, or any, series consider the overall condition of your health and be realistic about what is possible for you. You may need to choose just one or two poses depending on how you are feeling, both physically and emotionally. Check with your healthcare professional and be wise about your choices for activity and exercise. You may want to ask about the appropriateness of Restorative Yoga for your specific condition. Always practice Restorative Yoga with awareness.

If a pose is painful, make whatever adjustment is needed. Take time to find whatever position brings comfort and relax for 10-15 minutes. If you cannot find a comfortable posture, stop and try Restorative Yoga again another day.

When you are ready to practice this series, take a few minutes to tune into the sensations in the body and recognize where tension is being held. Let the breath be a guide to deep awareness of the body/mind in the present moment. Remember to surrender to whatever arises in each moment without trying to control or manipulate. Let each pose unfold.

(1) Supported Half-Dog Pose

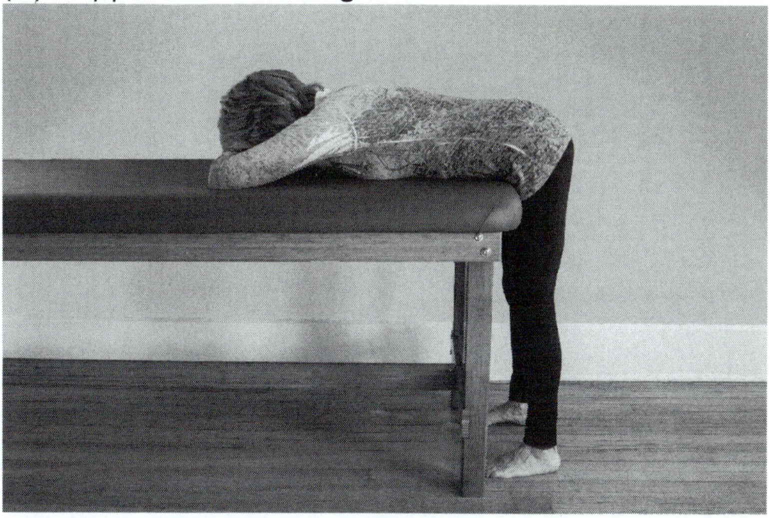

Props:

Table
1 or more single-fold blankets

Time:

2-3 minutes

Benefits:

Releases tension in the back
Stretches muscles along the spine
Relieves stiffness in the lower back

Cautions:

Take off your socks so as to not slide
Be extra careful not to exacerbate any back condition
If you feel pain as you bend forward, stop the pose

This pose requires the use of a table over which you will bend forward and rest your torso. It is important that your body is at a 90-degree angle in order to bring the lower back into gentle traction and stretch the long back muscles. Be sure to have your feet hip-distance apart and directly under the hip sockets.

Step close enough to the table so it is lightly touching the tops of your legs. Bend forward from the point where your torso meets the legs. If you are not at a right angle as you come to rest on the table, take time to adjust the height by adding one or more folded blankets.

As you fold forward observe how the torso lengthens and the back of the body stretches. Let your arms rest on the table, stretching alongside the head. You may prefer to fold the arms at the elbows and rest the side of your head on them. Be certain to turn your head to the other side halfway through the time you remain in the pose.

Breathe effortlessly ~ slow and easy. Let the torso and arms soften into the table. With your knees slightly bent, allow the weight of your legs to drop toward the earth. Fill the body with breath as you inhale. Feel spacious inside your body. Notice the neck and back lengthen with each exhalation. You only need stay in the posture for 2-3 minutes.

Take your time coming out of this pose. Keeping your knees slightly bent, use your arms to lift the torso off the props and stand in a relaxed position next to the table. Stand for a few moments (at least 5 complete breaths) before moving to the next posture.

Half-Dog Pose provides a simple way to traction your lower back. The muscles along the spine release while the pelvis is stabilized and the legs are grounded. For those who are unable to do the full version of Downward Dog, this is a great way to receive its benefits. Enjoy the relief in your lower back.

(2) Supported Fish Pose

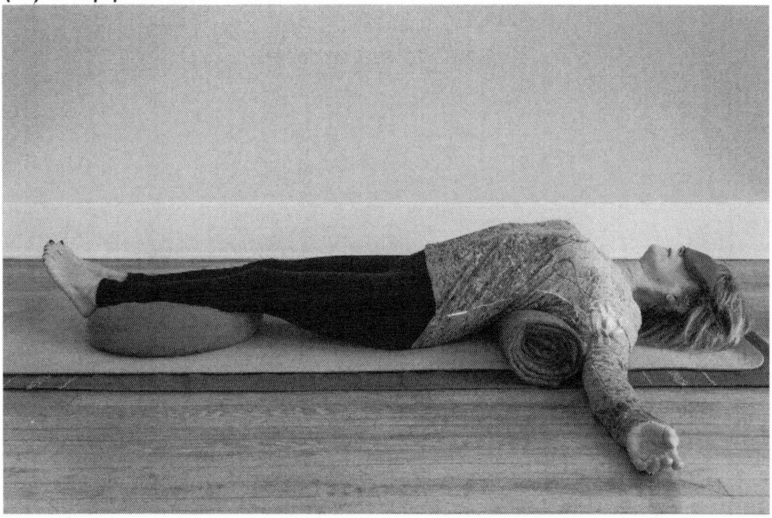

Props:
- Rolled blanket or bolster
- Zafu
- Rolled towel or small neck pillow
- Eye bag

Time:
- 1-3 minutes

Benefits:
- Counter pose for rounded spine
- Energizes the front body
- Stimulates the internal organs
- Lengthens the spine
- Deep muscular stretch of the back

Cautions: Do not practice if ~
- You have pain as you lie in the pose
- You have diagnosed disc disease
- You are more than 3 months pregnant

This gentle backbend gives your body welcome relief from the normal way the body is held with rounded shoulders and collapsed chest. It is a very useful counter pose.

Almost all of us experience back pain at some point in our lives. It is helpful to know some simple, gentle low-stress techniques to encourage healing. *Supported Fish Pose* is a gentle introduction to backbends for those who have a tender lower back.

To come into this position in a safe way, lie down on one side of your body and roll onto a rolled blanket or bolster. (See page 16 for more details) Adjust your body so a slight arch in the upper back is felt and the breath remains smooth and easy. If the upper back is uncomfortable or the arch can barely be felt, the rolled blanket can be adjusted by unrolling it until a comfortable arch is formed in the upper back. If a deeper backbend is appropriate, switch to a bolster. Place another cushion or zafu under the knees to relieve any discomfort in your lower back.

Feel the breath and follow its slow, even rhythm. As the mind rests in the breath, the body softens. Become aware of places that may be tense or tight and places where the breath flows easily.

Notice the arms wide and free. With each inhalation, the front body opens. With the exhalation, the belly and internal organs soften and the mind quiets. Allow the back to sink deeper into the props. As the back body releases, feel the pelvis soften and the hip sockets become spacious. The legs become heavy and the feet flop open about hip-width apart.

Remain in this position for 1-3 minutes to begin. If you are comfortable, stay in this gentle backbend for as long as your schedule allows. You may find that you want to set a timer so you don't fall asleep. As the pose completes itself, gradually bring awareness into the body. Take your time coming back. Begin to move slowly rolling onto the right side and resting briefly before coming to a seated position.

(3) Elevated Twist on a Bolster Pose

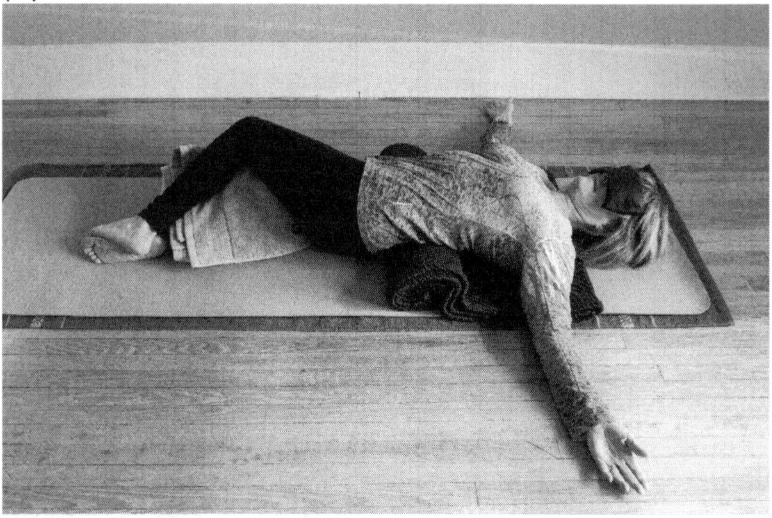

Props:

Rolled blanket or bolster
Rolled towel or pillow between legs
Eye bag

Time:

1-3 minutes on each side

Benefits:

Stretches the muscles holding pelvis and trunk
Opens the chest and lungs
Stimulates the kidneys
Stretches the small muscles of the spine
Brings low back into traction relieving discs
Enhances overall health of the spine

Cautions: Do not practice if ~

You have hiatal hernia or heart problems
You are more than 3 months pregnant

This pose offers a gentle, but invigorating way to stretch the external rotator muscles found deep in the outer hips. The muscles of the side waist and rib cage are also lengthened and the sacral-lumbar spine receives a gentle twist.

Sit in the middle of the bolster or blanket roll. Bend your knees and place your feet on the mat. Allow your hands to support you as you slide down onto the support so that your buttock rests on the bolster and your shoulders are on the floor. Press your feet into the floor and lift your hips so that you can move them as far to the left as possible. As the knees drop to the right toward the floor let your feet align with the hips. Check to see that the lowest rib on either side of your back is supported by the prop. Let the arms rest at the "T" position with your palms up. If this is too much, find the appropriate height by unrolling the blanket or switching the bolster for a blanket.

Place a pillow or towel between your knees and perhaps another towel under the bottom knee if needed. Slowly bring the knees up toward the chest, one at a time, until they are at a 90-degree angle. Let your pelvis roll over so that you are lying on your right side. If the left shoulder lifts off the floor, do not force it down. Stretch through the left arm and hand and if needed, add another towel or small pillow to support the shoulder.

In this pose, the back is slightly arched. Make certain your chest is open and the back has a slight arch by lifting the breastbone as you gently press the tailbone down. Be sure your body is comfortable even though it is in this twisted position.

Focus on the gentle twists created by the props and allow the breath to come into a smooth, deep and natural flow. Notice the stretch in your shoulder and the stretch caused by the knees dropping to the opposite side. Come into a balance between these and enjoy the opening in the chest and along the pectoral muscles. Feel the stretch in the outer hip. Bringing flexibility to these muscles is important to the health of your lower back.

Stay in the position for about a minute and gradually increase the time as you practice this pose. Bring your awareness into the present moment with each breath. Allow the inhalation to expand your body from the inside and completely soften and let go with each exhale. To come out of the pose, roll on to your back and lift your legs one at a time. Lower your feet to the floor and rest for several breaths.

When you are ready, repeat on the left side. Remember one side may feel different from the other. Gently move into the pose only to the point where you feel the stretch without any discomfort or pain. Remain in the pose for one minute, being present with each breath and allowing the pose to slowly deepen. Slide off the bolster or rolled blanket in the direction of your head and come onto your side. Stay curled up and take several long, easy breaths before returning to a seated position.

This posture is an excellent remedy for your lower back. It not only stretches the small muscles of the spine, but also tractions the lower back and releases tension in the discs between the vertebrae. The muscles that hold the pelvis and trunk together receive a deep stretch. Additionally, this twist opens your lungs, chest, and diaphragm improving your breathing. Thus your overall well-being is enhanced.

(4) Supported Child's Pose

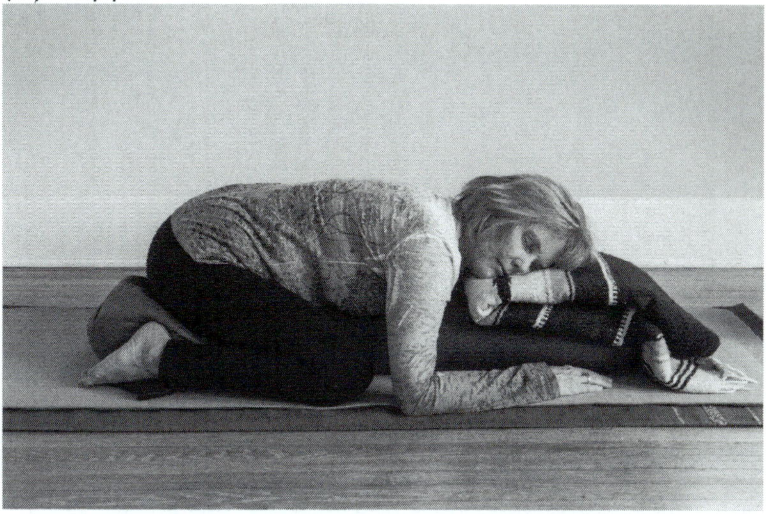

Props:

Bolster
Zafu
2 or more blankets

Time:

2-4 minutes

Benefits:

Stretches the lower back
Opens the back body
Relieves tension in the shoulders
Quiets the mind
Brings a sense of feeling safe and serene

Cautions:

Protect knees, ankles and feet
Limit practice if you have a severe back condition
Do not do this pose if more than 3 months pregnant

If your back aches from sitting or standing, this pose will be very helpful. Following the last two postures, *Supported Child's Pose* offers a time to fold forward and counter the gentle backbends you have just finished.

To prepare, come onto all fours. Feel the flow of the breath moving through the body. Stay with the feelings and sensations in the body/mind. Relax the hips back toward the heels and separate the knees, allow the big toes to move toward one another and possibly touch. Slide a bolster or stack of 2-3 blankets vertically between the legs and let the torso soften onto the prop. Support the head with 1-2 folded blankets or towels so that the head rests comfortably on the right cheek. (Halfway through the pose turn and rest on the left cheek.)

Allow the body to find a position where your arms are resting comfortably. Slip a pillow or zafu in the space between the buttocks and the heels. Lift your hips slightly to allow the placement of the cushion and then feel the pelvis melt into the support.

Once you are comfortable, tune into your breath and feel it move into your back. With each inhale notice the shoulders and upper back expand. As you exhale let your hips and tailbone release toward the floor as your entire back expands and softens. Let the breath flow through your body like a wave and enjoy this safe and supported posture.

After 2-3 minutes (halfway through the pose), turn your head and rest on the opposite cheek. Let the support cradle the head so the shoulders can release. Feel the heart melting into the bolster and soften the belly. Allow the world to dissolve as awareness draws inward toward the center of being. With every muscle, bone, organ, tissue and cell softening, surrender to that deep ocean of tranquility. Let the pose nurture your back and bring relief to tired and sore back muscles.

Remember to change the position of your head halfway through the time you spend in the pose. Allow at least 4-6 minutes in this pose and when you feel complete, come out by using the strength of your arms to lift your body off of the props. Find your way into a seated position and rest until ready to move on to the final position.

(5) Shavasana with Legs on a Chair

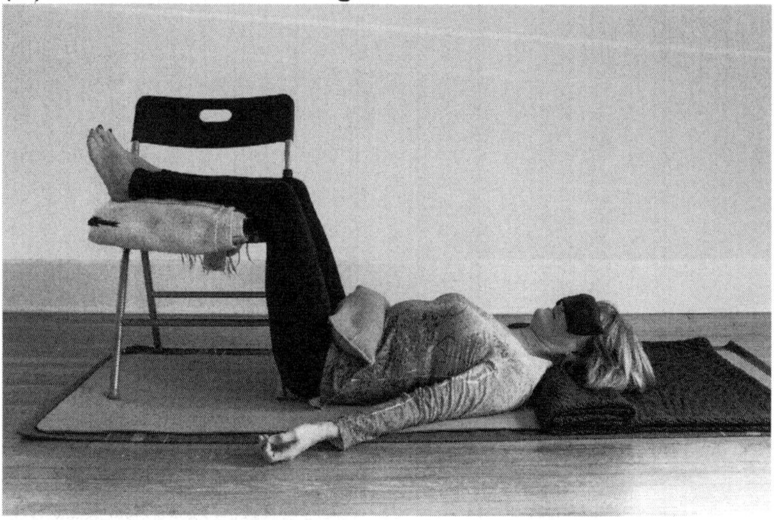

Props:

- Chair
- 2 blankets
- Eye bag
- Sandbag (optional)

Time:

- 5-10 minutes

Benefits:

- Releases muscles of lower back
- Revives the legs
- Relaxes the abdominal organs and muscles
- Reduces fatigue
- Slows the heart rate
- Increases inwardness

Cautions:

- Move slowly and deliberately as you come out
- Avoid this if you are more than 3 months pregnant

This variation of *Shavasana* provides a deep release in the lower back. In addition to a chair, you may use a sandbag or firm pillow to release the abdominal muscles. This combination of chair for the legs and sandbag for the belly will result in maximum relief to the lower back.

Prepare for this pose by placing a standard fold blanket on the chair in front of you and a single fold, rolled blanket positioned to cradle your head. If you use a chair with a cushioned seat, you may not need the blanket. Use your hands and arms to brace yourself as you lie back onto the blankets. Bring your legs up on the chair so that the knees and hips are bent. They should form a right angle.

If your legs are not comfortable, you may need to add one or more blankets in order to lift your torso. Remember to take time to adjust the props in order to relax.

The blanket for under your head should be rolled once or twice to support the curve of your neck. As your head rests on the blanket, your chin should be slightly lower than the forehead. This position allows the mind to quiet.

Now place the sandbag or a firm pillow across your belly. Cover your eyes with the eye bag and let the eyes soften their inner gaze toward the heart. Allow the arms to rest a comfortable distance from the sides of your body with palms up.

Begin to notice your breath. Once it is even, release tension in your body through a progressive relaxation procedure. With your head resting softly on the support notice all the sensations inside the month, tongue, teeth, upper and lower palate. Relax the jaw. Soften the face and eyes. Let the eyes rest back into the sockets.

Move into the neck and throat releasing any constriction or tightness. Proceed to move your awareness through the body noticing the shoulders, the arms, the hands and fingers. Feel the chest and upper back sink into the props. Let all the internal organs bathe in the breath as it flows in and out of the body.

Feel the hips, pelvis, lower back and sacrum all soften as the soothing rhythm of the breath continues. Let the legs be heavy and the feet float on the chair.

Remain in this pose for at least 5-10 minutes. If you would like, you may remain for 15-20 minutes. The pose is complete when you no longer feel the weight of the sandbag. Slide the sandbag (or pillow) off to one side and take several breaths. Roll to one side, letting the eye bag slide off the eyes and then use your arms to help you sit up.

Move slowly and deliberately back into your day. Notice the openness and relief in the lower back and belly. Remember to take time to repeat these poses whenever the chronic pain returns.

Self-care
is often overlooked
as we busy ourselves
with limitless activities.

Take time
to pamper yourself
and you will be gifted
with radiant health and well being.

Chapter 5

Deepen Your Breathing

If it is only health you want, breathe.
If you are in need of a strong immune system, breathe.
If emotional and mental health is your desire, breathe.
If you...wish to truly know your divine nature, then breathe.
~ Richard Miller, Ph.D.

There are several poses that bring awareness to the process of breathing. Awareness allows us to change old patterns and develop habits that encourage full, deep, and comfortable breathing.

The Deepen Your Breathing practice is beneficial for everyone. The poses open the chest, increase flexibility in the ribcage, and expand limited breathing functions caused by anxiety, fear or other emotional tightness in the body/mind. For those who have nasal congestion due to allergies, asthma or flu, this series helps increase capacity in the lungs, enabling more complete exhalations and deeper inhalations.

Yoga postures and breathing techniques have long been known to increase lung capacity. In fact, they help the entire respiratory system function more efficiently. They can actually counter the shrinking that occurs in the ribcage as we age.

Improving the breath involves several structures in the torso:

- the diaphragm
- the intercostal muscles
- the ribcage
- the mid-back
- the pectoral muscles
- the shoulder girdle

The diaphragm, the major muscle of respiration, is often constricted by our posture. The intercostal muscles connect the ribs and can become very tight and immobile, unless they are consciously stretched. Both the diaphragm and intercostal muscles must have space to expand and contract. When working properly these muscles lift the ribs on the inhale and allow the ribs to drop on the exhale.

The thoracic spine in the mid-back also needs to be flexible in order for our respiration to be efficient. The pectoral muscles found at the top of the chest help the shoulder girdle expand and broaden. This affects how deeply we can breathe. Tight pectoral muscles cause the shoulders to roll inward and the breastbone to drop. This collapsing of the chest limits three movements necessary for proper breathing:

1) movement of the thoracic spine,
2) expanding of intercostal muscles and
3) movement of the diaphragm.

This series begins with *Supported Crescent Moon Pose* to open the side body. Then *Gently Flowing Brook Pose* opens the lungs and stretches the diaphragm and intercostal muscles. *Supported Tranquility Pose,* a modified inversion, lifts the ribcage, opens the lungs, and helps release any unneeded fluid from the chest. *Supported Heroine/Hero Pose* lifts the diaphragm off the abdominal organs and opens the throat and chest.

The series ends with a variation of *Shavasana* that quiets the mind, encourages a smooth breath to move through the lungs, and allows the diaphragm to expand and contract with ease. All poses support breathing to become easier, smoother, deeper and more effortless.

(1) Supported Crescent Moon (Side Bending)

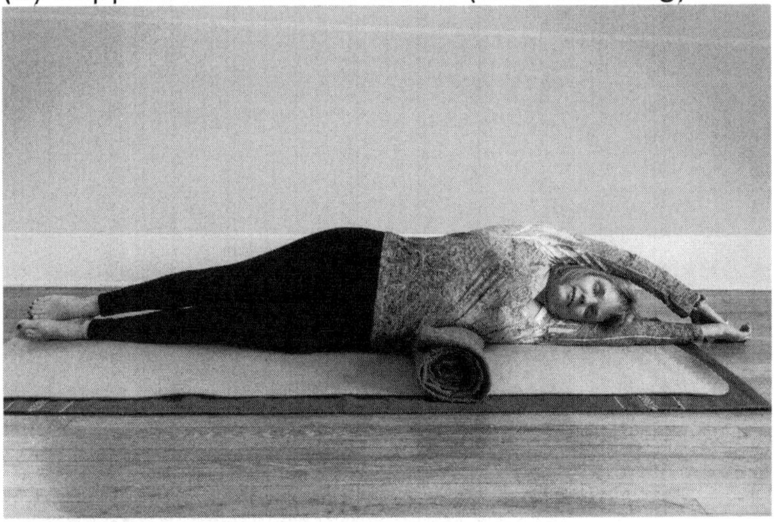

Props:

Bolster or rolled blanket
Eye bag
Small rolled towel, if needed

Time:

1-2 minutes on each side

Benefits:

Stretches the side body
Stimulates internal organs
Improves respiration
Relieves stress and anxiety

Cautions:

Be careful not to overstretch
Be certain to support your neck

Side-stretching poses lengthen the muscles between the ribs and pelvis, including the area of the low back. They open the sides of the rib cage, improving rib cage mobility and the expansiveness of the lungs. When the arm stretches overhead, the large muscle extending from the back waist to the armpit also stretches. The result is easier breathing in all situations, including Yoga, Pranayama (breathing techniques), and aerobic activities.

Supported Crescent Moon Pose brings a welcome stretch to the side body and extends the spine laterally. A rolled blanket, or bolster, is placed horizontally at the edge of the right hip. Bend your knees and slowly bring the right side of your body to rest just above the waist on the blanket or bolster. With the right arm outstretched, rest the back of the hand on the floor as the side of your head nestles into your upper arm.

If the neck is uncomfortable, place a rolled towel or small pillow between it and your arm. If the stretch is too much, adjust the bolster or exchange it for a rolled blanket. Always tune into how the body feels before continuing. Bring the left arm overhead and let the palms come together in prayer position. Feel the entire left side of the body stretch and open.

Allow the breath to move into the torso and expand the left side body. With each breath, notice the opening between the ribs increase and allow any places of tension or tightness to dissolve. After 1-2 minutes, let the top arm float to your side as you exhale. Slowly lift the upper body and move to the other side.

Take time to adjust the body, coming to rest on the left side. With the left arm resting on the floor, let the head settle into the upper arm. Check to see if your neck is comfortable. Bring the right arm up and over alongside the ear with your hands in prayer position above your head and resting on the floor. Breathe into the stretch and feel the right side of the body open. Relax into the posture as the breath becomes more effortless.

Full complete exhalations allow the body to release unwanted toxins from the cells of the body and to bring more oxygen and nutrients into the body with the inhalation.

Lateral poses give attention to an overlooked part of the torso. They stimulate the internal organs, elongate the side body, and bring oxygen into this part of the body. They help relieve stress and anxiety as the torso opens.

The crescent moon
reminds us every little sliver of
our being is filled with radiant light and love.
Be the light you are...

2) Gently Flowing Pose

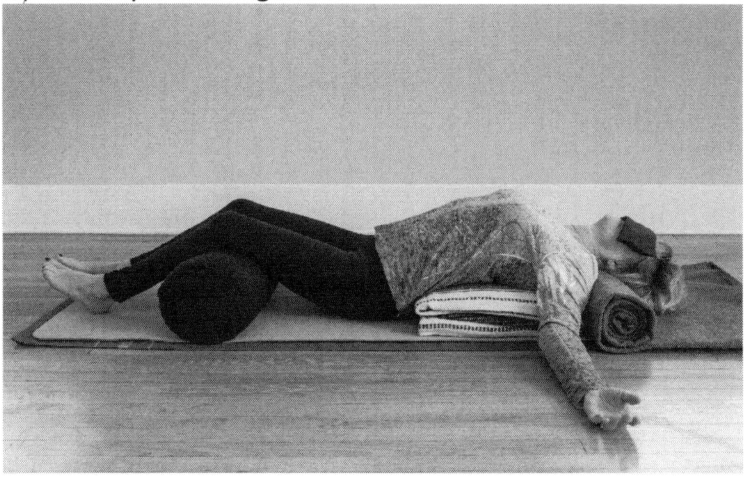

Props:

Rolled blanket or bolster
2 single-fold blankets
Long-roll blanket
Eye bag

Time:

3-5 minutes

Benefits:

Opens the chest and lungs
Reduces fatigue
Improves digestion
Lifts your spirits

Cautions:

Check with health provider if you have spinal problems or disc disease.
Skip less if you are more than 3 months pregnant

Just as water gently flows over rocks, your body gently flows over the props in this pose giving the front body a way to open. Three areas (the throat, heart and belly) may need to be released in order to deepen your breath. The support under the neck gently opens your throat, the blankets open your chest, and the zafu or bolster under the knees protects your lower back and allows the belly to relax.

As you prepare for this pose, you may need to try differing heights of blankets. Start with two stacked blankets. If this is too much of a lift for the upper back remove one blanket. Lie down at the midpoint of the blanket so that the shoulder blades are supported. Once the correct height is determined, sit up and arrange the other props. The bolster or zafu can be placed under the knees and the long-roll blanket above the stack of blankets to support the neck.

Take your time as you gently lie down over the three supports. Once the body is comfortable, make certain the arch of the neck is supported and your head tilts back gently. The throat should be open and relaxed. The bolster under your knees comforts your lower back. Bring your arms into a "T" position, if possible. If you feel even a slight degree of discomfort, roll to one side, slowly sit up, and rearrange the props in whatever way necessary. It is crucial that your neck is completely relaxed.

Place an eye bag over your eyes and begin to notice your breath. Feel the touch of the breath as it flows into the nostrils, down the throat and fills the lungs. Let the belly fill as the inhalation completes itself and then notice how the belly softens into the props as you exhale.

With the lips slightly parted and your tongue floating in the mouth, swallow and release any tension in the throat. Feel the skin of the face melting and the cheeks hollow. Notice the throat opening to allow more air into your lungs.

Bring attention to your heart and notice how supported you are, not only physically, but emotionally as well. Allow whatever feelings are present to simply arise and be there without trying to name them. Imagine the breath flowing in and out of the heart, and feel what is present as each moment unfolds. Some students notice sadness, tightness, or constriction; while others feel loving kindness, compassion, joy or vast spaciousness. Whatever is present, be the observer without wanting to either attach or detach from it.

Move your awareness into the belly and notice how it softens into the spine with each exhalation. With the inhalation feel how it expands, the breath moving gently into all the nooks and crannies of the belly. Let the belly continue to expand and soften with each breath until it is spacious and open. Enjoy the deep, safe sense of openness in your throat, heart and belly.

Stay in this pose for 3-5 minutes. Let the body finds its way into a full, deep breathing pattern. Enjoy the emotional release as the body also lets go of tension. Begin to move and slowly find your way back. Stretch and become fully present in your body. Roll to the right side, rest briefly and return to a seated position.

(3) Supported Tranquility Pose

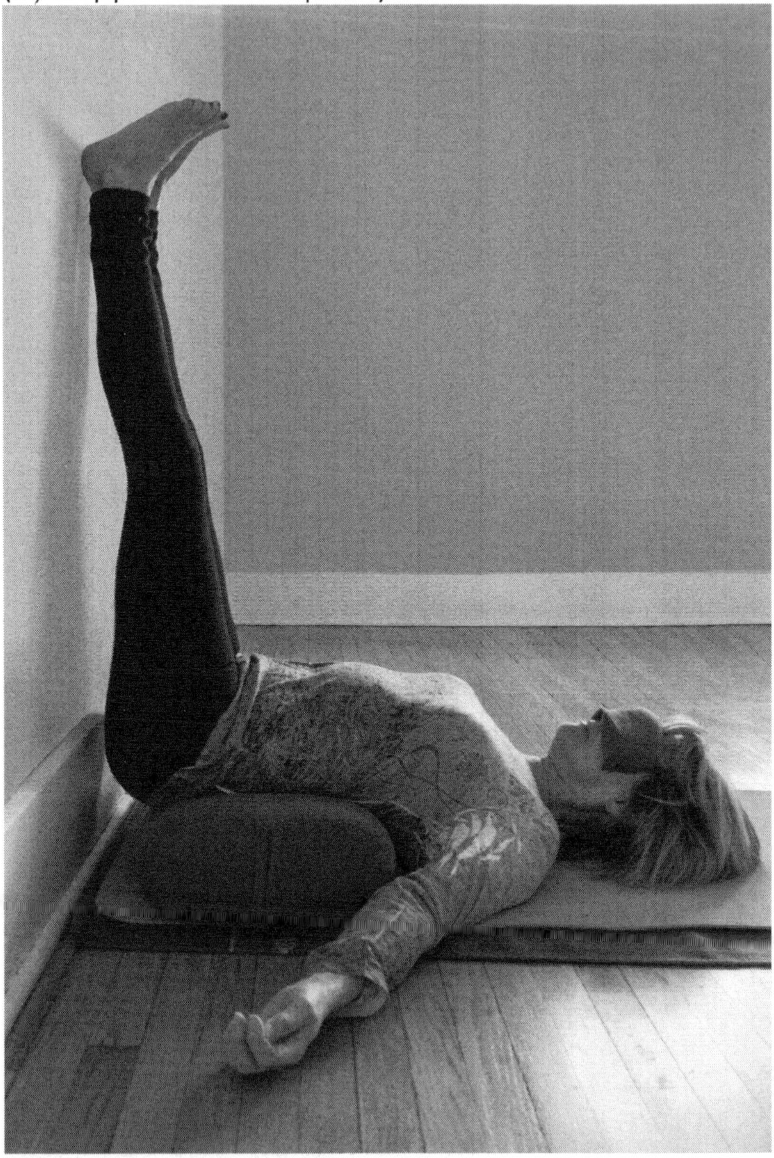

Props:

Bolster or zafu
1 or more folded blankets or towels
Eye bag

Time:

7-10 minutes

Benefits:

Enhances the breathing process
Restores tired legs and feet
Soothes the nervous system
Quiets the mind
Reenergizes both physically and emotionally
Balances blood pressure
Reduces fatigue

Cautions:

If there is discomfort in the back, bend the knees, place your feet on a wall or loosely cross your ankles and let the wall support you.

Not recommended for those who have hiatal hernia, eye pressure, retinal problems, heart condition, neck injury or are menstruating.

If this pose creates pressure in the head, do not do it.

Supported Tranquility Pose is a gentle inversion in which the pelvis and torso rest in a slight backbend and the legs hang above the heart. Legs may rest against a wall or just extend into the air above the hips. (See p.

103) As in all inversions, gravity plays a big part in reversing the usual position of the body in space.

One visualization to consider during this pose is that of a waterfall cascading down the legs into pools created by the shape of the belly and gently overflowing into the chest.

To prepare for this pose, sit with the right side of the body against the wall and place a support next to the left hip. Come onto the floor and swing the legs up onto the wall. The sitting bones should be as close to the wall as comfortable. The tighter the hamstrings, the more space may be needed between the wall and the body.

Once the legs are on the wall, bend the knees and press the soles of the feet into the wall to elevate the hips. Slide the cushion under and rest back on the support. Make whatever adjustments necessary to be comfortable.

If you prefer, you may try a variation that does not use the wall as a support. Lie on your back with knees bent and feet close to the hips. Press your feet into the floor allowing the hips to lift, slide a zafu or bolster under the hips and let them sink into the support. Make certain hips and pelvis are completely at ease.

Slowly feel the legs reach upward until they are hanging in the air above the hips. It is important they are directly above the hips in order for gravity to draw the top of the leg into the hip socket. The perfect placement is found when your legs rest in the air without muscular tension. The weight of the legs release both the hip joints and the lower back.

Remember the position of your neck is important. If there is any strain or if the chin feels it is pressing into your chest, use a small rolled towel or neck pillow to support it. The prop should support the vertebra (C7) at the base of the neck near the shoulders, and not be placed in the center of the neck where the curve is the greatest.

With the focus on improving respiration, let the breath flow smooth and even. Keep your attention on the chest and notice how the ribcage and entire chest cavity expand with each in-breath. Feel fatigue and tension drain from the body as you exhale.

You may practice this posture for 7-10 minutes. When your body is ready, begin the process of returning to an upright position with deliberate attention. If your legs are hanging in the air without support of a wall, bring the feet to your mat, hip distance apart. If you are at the wall, place your feet on it with your knees bent. Press the feet into the floor or the wall, as appropriate, and lift the hips just enough to remove the support. Slowly bring the hips back to the floor and roll to one side keeping the body curled in a fetal position. Take a breath or two before coming to a seated position. Remember to use your arms to lift the torso so that you do not strain your lower back.

Along with helping relieve breathing problems, this pose serves as an antidote for the systemic effects of stress. Regular practice brings an overall sense of wellbeing.

(4) Supported Hero/Heroine Pose

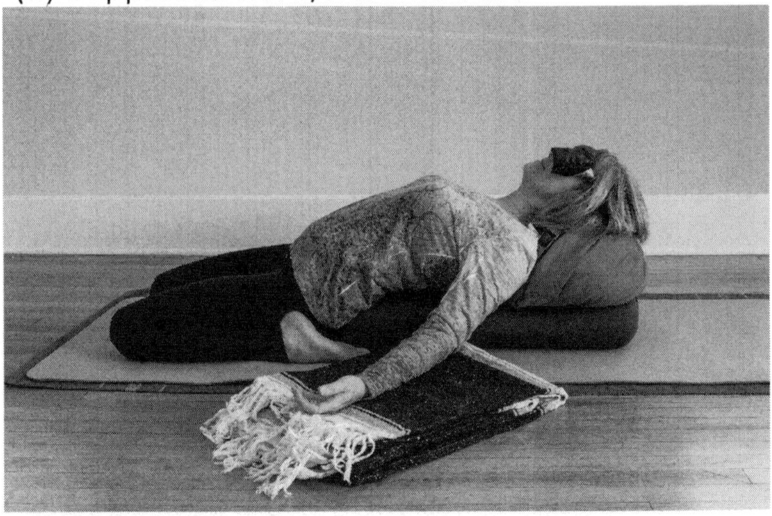

Props:

- Bolster
- 3 or more folded blankets
- Eye bag
- Rolled towel(s)

Time:

- 3-4 minutes to begin; up to 10 minutes

Benefits:

- Opens the throat, bronchial tubes and lungs
- Relieves pressure in sinus areas of head
- Reduces fatigue in legs
- Stretches the ankles, front of the feet and toes
- Lifts diaphragm off of stomach and liver (relieving indigestion and nausea)

Cautions:

Use a rolled washcloth or eye bag under the ankle to relieve discomfort in the feet or ankles.

If there is discomfort in the quadriceps, use another blanket under the spine for support.

Supported Hero/Heroine Pose can be beneficial if you are congested and want your breathing to deepen as you relax. It helps reduce anxiety and emotional distress by opening the lungs and allowing the amount of air you breathe to increase.

Many conditions, such as asthma or bronchitis, result in shallow breathing. This causes a buildup of carbon dioxide in the bloodstream and can lead to increased feelings of anxiety.

To prepare, make certain you are comfortable in the seated variation of Hero's Pose. From a kneeling position, sit back between your heels. If there is any discomfort, sit on a folded blanket or block placed between your feet. You may need to return to kneeling and gently move the calf muscles toward the heels and hold them as you sit back onto the support again.

These adjustments should relieve any pressure on the knees, ankles and feet. To diminish discomfort on the tops of the feet use a rolled towel or eye bag under each ankle. It is important to note the position of the feet. They need to be in alignment with the knees and pointing straight back.

Once you are comfortable, place a bolster long ways (vertically) behind you and add a zafu or folded blanket at the far end to support your head. Slowly using your hands for support lie back on the props. If your head needs more support, add another blanket or small pillow. Make certain your chest is open and your abdomen is comfortable. You should be at a 45-degree angle to the floor.

Take time to find the most comfortable position, resting on the supports. Your knees can be as far apart as needed for comfort. Check to see that your knees are aligned with your feet, toes straight back. Turning the foot out strains the inner knee and may cause discomfort.

Take two more folded blankets and place one under each arm for additional comfort and support. With your eye bag over the eyes, give yourself permission to let go. Feel the legs and hips become heavy and the chest lift with each breath. As you inhale, notice the chest expands horizontally. As you exhale, visualize the chest remaining in this new expanded position. Let the chest continue to open with each cycle of breath.

If you begin to gasp for breath, let go of all effort and find your breath's natural rhythm. Once you are comfortable again, observe the upper chest as it expands. Each inhalation can stretch the chest cavity and open the entire respiratory system. Welcome each breath, allow your breathing to be slow, easy and natural. To begin, remain in this pose 3-4 minutes. Once the body is more accustomed to *Supported Heroine Pose*, the time may be increased to 5-10 minutes.

Return to a seated position by using your arms to lift the torso. Either release each leg and bring them around in front of you or come on to your hands and knees. Stretch the legs before standing and take care to move slowly and deliberately.

(5) Shavasana Pose with Elevated Chest

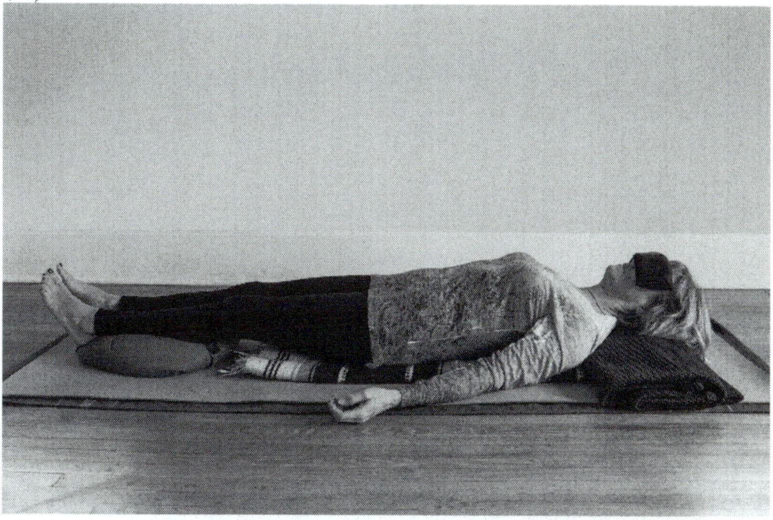

Props:

- 2 folded or rolled blankets
- Long-roll blanket
- Eye bag

Time:

- 10-15 minutes

Benefits:

- Reduces fatigue and anxiety often accompanying respiratory difficulties
- Lowers blood pressure and heart rate
- Releases muscular tension
- Helps with chronic pain
- Enhances immune response
- Improves sleep

Cautions:

If more than 3 months pregnant, practice relaxation lying on the side of the torso.

This series ends with *Shavasana Pose with Elevated Chest,* a variation of *Shavasana Pose* in which the chest is elevated. It is an appropriate pose for you if you have any difficulty breathing in a lying down position. Breathing deeply is more accessible in this supported posture.

To prepare, you need three blankets. Place the first blanket long ways so that as you lie down the short end touches your tailbone. This blanket supports and lifts the chest slightly. The second blanket placed across the end of the first one (like a "T") supports the head and neck. The third blanket (zafu or bolster if you prefer) goes under the knees to allow the lower back to relax.

Let your body move onto the props and notice how you feel. Your head should be slightly higher than your chest and your chest should be higher than your abdomen. Place the eye bag on your eyes.

Notice the position of your arms and legs. They should be the same distance from the sides of your body. If the hands feel comfortable with your palms up, turn them to this position. It is a subtle signal to the brain to relax. Remember the most important thing is that your body/mind finds complete support and is at ease in this pose.

As you turn into your breath, imagine a smooth and easy flow. Whatever the difficulty might be, see your breath melting away all tension and discomfort. As you inhale, feel the natural expansion of the body. As you exhale, notice how effortless and easy breathing can be. Without striving, let the breath slowly wash over and through you.

After 10-15 minutes (or less, if you wish), begin to come back by slowly bending one knee and then the other. Feel the body move to one side as your eye bag slides off the eyes. Rest in this fetal position for a few breaths before coming back to a seated position. Remember to use your hands and the strength of your arms to come up. Take your time as you move back into your daily activities.

Breath is life.

Yoga
tells us
we are each given
a finite number of breaths for our lifetime.
When you deepen and lengthen your breath, you extend your lifespan by not using your breaths as quickly.

Restorative poses
help you increase your lung capacity.
The respiratory system opens and your lungs accept more breath. These poses, practiced regularly,
help develop the ability
to let go and
just BE.

Chapter 6

Soothe Aches and Pains

Be strong then, and enter into your body:
There you have a solid place for your feet.
Think about it carefully.
Don't go off somewhere else!
~Kabir

Many people hold tension in their physical bodies creating unwanted discomfort and chronic aches. Headaches and neck and shoulder pain are common ailments. The following postures can bring lasting relief when practiced consistently.

What is unique about this series is your intention to care for your specific pain through a series of supported poses and directed breathing techniques. If you have headaches, you may wish to wrap your head with an elastic band for each pose. For chronic shoulder or neck pain, you may want to include an herbal hot/cold pack to provide additional relief and comfort. Directing the breath to specific areas where tension is being held can bring a much appreciated release of tightness.

Using a head wrap applies pressure on the forehead, the temples, and the sinus areas. It prevents light from disturbing the eyes, a common contributor to headaches. Headache bands can be found online, in specialty medical supply shops, or you may purchase an Ace bandage from the local drugstore.

When you wrap your head be sure to cover the eyes and end with extra material that can be tucked in so that you are not resting on the bulge. Start at the base of the skull with the loose end held in place behind one ear. With your other hand slowly wrap the bandage over the opposite ear, crossing over one eye. Then bring the bandage down slightly to gently press around the head again. As the wrap makes its way to the front of the head a second time, wrap the other eye.

Check that the eyes and ears are covered and tuck the remainder wherever you wish. You won't want it to be at the back of the head because the bulge might be uncomfortable as you lie in the supine poses.

In between the poses fold the front portion of the wrap back so that you can see to set up the next pose. At the end of the series, remove the wrap slowly releasing the pressure gradually. This way you will maintain the comfort and relief you have found. Practice wrapping your head to avoid frustration with the bandage when you use it for these poses.

You also may want to use a neck or shoulder wrap. The neck, shoulder or back wraps can be placed in a variety of positions bringing relief to painful places in the body. These wraps can be warmed in the microwave or chilled in the freezer.

This series can include any of the poses from the standard practice, but these specific poses are offered here. First, *Supported Shavasana Pose with a Head Wrap* is considered a most important posture for relieving headaches. Next, try *Half-Dog Pose* to release the back, shoulders and neck. *Supported Bridge Pose* stretches the neck and upper back muscles and can relieve headaches and may prevent them. *Supported Tranquility Pose* offers a very effective way to relieve all over body aches and pains. *Supported Reclining Pose* completes this series and complements the other postures to bring relief to chronic pain and emotional or mental discomfort.

(1) Supported Shavasana Pose with Head Wrap

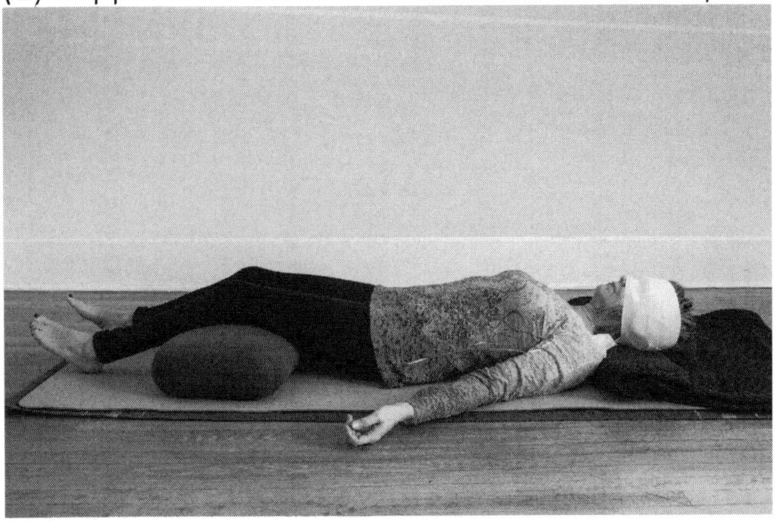

Props:
- Bolster or zafu
- Folded blanket
- Headache bandage wrap or option

Time:
- 10-20 minutes

Benefits:
- Releases muscular tension
- Slows heart rate
- Reduces fatigue
- Lowers blood pressure

Cautions:
- Do not practice if more than 3 months pregnant

Take time to wrap the head if you wish. Come into the supine position with supports under both the knees and the neck. Remember, *Supported Shavasana Pose* is considered by many to be the ultimate posture for relaxing body, mind, and spirit and offers an excellent way to relieve headaches. It brings a deep sense of calm and connection to those who faithfully practice it. If you have time for only one pose, this is the one to choose.

Settle into a lying down position, find the breath and allow it to move slowly through the body. Come into a deep sense of its rhythm. Fill and expand the body as you inhale. Soften and release all tension or discomfort on the exhale. Once the body has found equanimity, tune into the sensations that arise. Notice the mouth and all the sensations inside the mouth, the teeth, tongue, jaw and gums. Let the tongue relax; feel it all the way into the root of the tongue.

Soften the skin of the face and let the head rest back into the blanket beneath it. Feel the forehead soften under the wrap and notice the space inside the skull. It may feel as if the brain is floating.

Feel sensations in the ears. Let the ears become funnels of vibrant energy and be aware of the folds and valleys of the external ears. Notice the eyes and consciously allow them to rest deeply into the sockets. Feel the muscles around the eyes soften.

Let the radiance of the eyes flow in a stream of energy through the back of the head and down the neck until the sensations of the throat can be identified. Swallow and release any tightness and let this whole area soften.

Feel the torso and the center of the chest. Let sensations of energy fill the heart and radiate out through the entire torso. Continue moving through the body into the arms and hands; the belly; the backside of the body; the hips and pelvis; and into the legs, ankles, and feet.

Feel the body soften and let go into the vast spaciousness that you are.

Remain in this pose for at least ten minutes, or even longer if possible. Of all Yoga poses, this is the best remedy for headaches.

When you are ready to move into the next pose, remember to do so slowly and deliberately. First, gently remove the wrap from your head and feel the body stretch. Draw in one knee and then the other as you roll to one side. Come to a seated position using the strength of your arms.

(2) Supported Half -Dog Pose

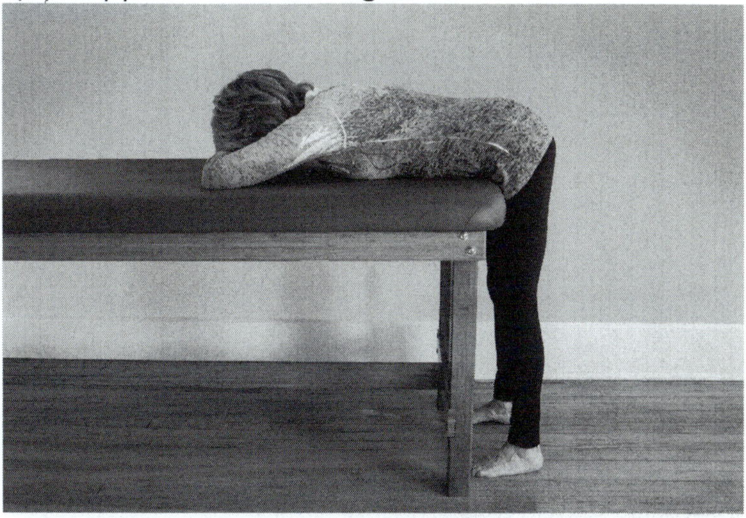

Props:

Table

1 or more single-fold blankets

Time:

2 minutes

Benefits:

Releases tension in the back

Stretches muscles along the spine

Relieves stiffness in the lower back

Cautions:

Take off your socks so as to not slide.

Be extra careful not to exacerbate any back condition. If you feel pain as you bend forward, skip this pose.

This pose requires the use of a table over which you will bend forward and rest your torso. It is important that your body is at a 90-degree angle in order to bring the lower back into a gentle traction and stretch the long muscles of the back. Be sure to have your feet hip-distance apart and directly under the hip sockets.

Step close enough to the table so it is lightly touching the tops of your legs. Bend forward from the point where your torso meets the legs. If you are not at a right angle as you come to rest on the table, take time to adjust the height by adding one or more folded blankets.

Adjust the elastic bandage if you are using one and cover your eyes. As you fold forward observe how the torso lengthens and the back body stretches. Let your arms rest on the table, stretching alongside the head. You may wish to fold the arms at the elbows and rest the side of your head on them. Be certain to turn your head to the other side halfway through the pose. To relax the neck and back further, you may want to ask someone to add a warm neck or back wrap once you are folded over the table.

Breathe effortlessly ~ slow and easy. Let the torso and arms soften into the table. With the knees slightly bent, allow the weight of your legs to drop toward the earth. Fill the body with breath as you inhale. Feel spaciousness inside your body. Notice the neck and back lengthen with each exhalation. You need only stay in the posture for 2-3 minutes.

Take your time coming out of this pose. Keeping your knees slightly bent, use your arms to lift the torso off the props and stand in a relaxed position next to the table. Stand for a few moments (at least 5 complete breaths) before moving to the next posture.

Half-Dog Pose provides a simple way to traction your lower back. The muscles along the spine release while the pelvis is stabilized and the legs are grounded. You might want to try to stretch a bit more by taking one or two steps back away from the table. Be aware of your body and do not overdo. If this pose intensifies your headache, eliminate it from the series.

(3) Supported Bridge Pose

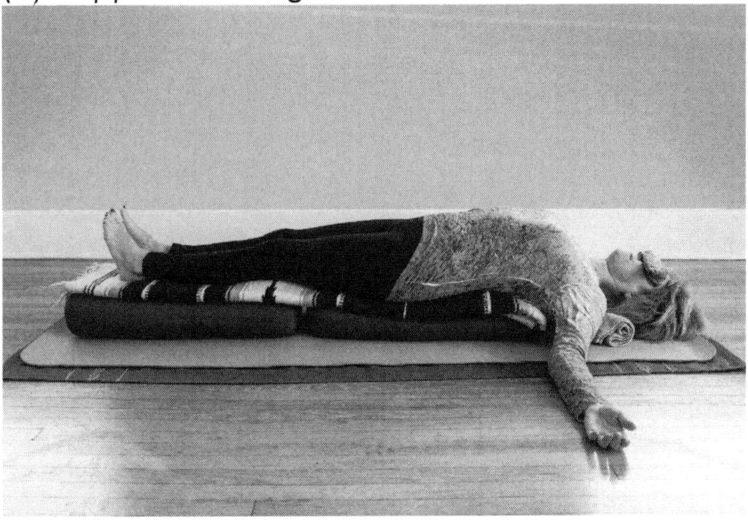

Props:

- 2 bolsters
- 1 or more blankets
- Rolled towel or neck pillow (optional)
- Eye bag

Time:

- 5-15 minutes

Benefits:

- Opens and releases the neck
- Releases pressure on the head
- Encourages breathing and helps reduce stress

Cautions:

Not recommended for those who should avoid inversions.

If there pose creates pressure in the head, do not do it.

> Avoid if you have any respiratory or sinus infections.
> Consult your health care professional, if you have concerns.

Place the bolsters end-to-end so your body fits on them. If your back is tight, you may want to start with a stack of blankets that is shorter than the bolsters. Standard bolsters are nine inches high. A stack of 2-3 folded blankets has a height of approximately six inches. In addition to the height of the props, it is important they support the length of the body and are uniform in height.

Straddle the props and lie back using your arms to lower yourself. Slide so your head, neck and shoulders rest on the floor, while the rest of your body remains on the bolsters. If you feel any discomfort, make the necessary adjustments. Bend your knees if there is tension in your lower back. Your feet can be on the bolsters or on the floor at each side of the support.

It is important to maintain the natural curve of your neck. If your chin is pressing into your chest, you may need to place a rolled towel under the neck where it meets the shoulders. This is critical to protect vertebra (C7). The towel should not be under the middle of the neck, but at its base. Try different ways of rolling the towel to find the most comfortable. You may not need the entire towel rolled; the part you don't roll can be under your head. You also might want to try a thin neck wrap that has been warmed.

If you are practicing to relieve a headache, you may wish to use an elastic bandage and cover the eyes. If you would rather use a warm or cool wrap, proceed with setting that up. Once you are ready, let the arms rest a comfortable distance away from your body.

Supported Bridge Pose helps to counter the habitual posture of having the head forward rather than in line with the shoulders. It releases the muscles at the back and sides of the neck. Tightness in these muscles are often responsible for head, neck and shoulder pain.

Take the next few moments to relax the eyes and soften your brow. Swallow and release the jaw and tongue. Notice sensations in the mouth and ears. Allow the muscles of the face, scalp and neck to soften and release any remaining tension. Feel the flow of your breath as it fills the chest. Let the ribs expand on the inhale and soften on the exhale. Move the breath into the places that are tight, tense or uncomfortable. Feel the spaces become open, allowing the tension to dissolve with each exhale.

Remain in the pose for as long as you are comfortable, 5-15 minutes. When ready, remove the eye bag or other prop from your eyes and slowly begin to slide off the bolsters or blankets so your head comes off the supports first. Let the entire torso rest on the floor, while your calves remain on the bolsters. Take several slow breaths. Then roll to one side, using your arms to press back into a seated position.

(4) Tranquility Pose at the Wall

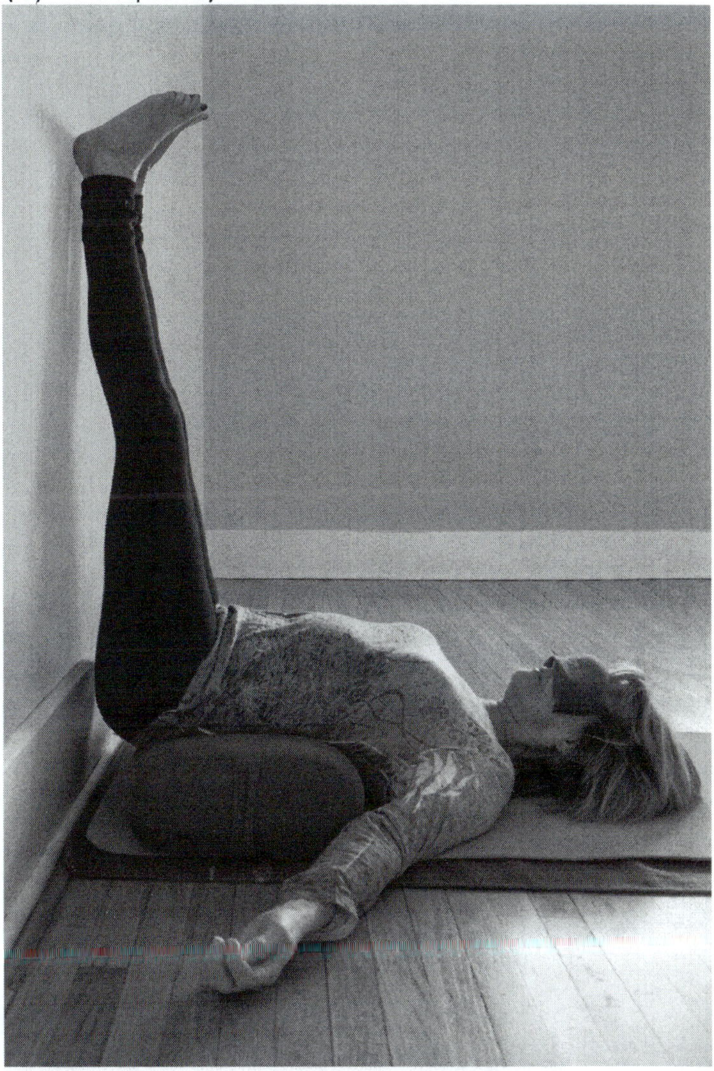

Props:

- Bolster or zafu
- 1 or more folded blankets or towels
- Eye bag

Time:

5-10 minutes

Benefits:

Restores tired legs and feet
Soothes the nervous system
Quiets the mind
Relieves headaches
Balances blood pressure
Regulates the thyroid gland

Cautions:

If any back discomfort, bend the knees, place your feet on a wall or loosely cross your ankles and let the wall support you.

Not recommended for those who should avoid inversions, if you have hiatal hernia, eye pressure, retinal problems, heart condition, neck injury or are menstruating.

If there is pressure in the head, do not do this.

In this variation of *Tranquility Pose,* you elevate the hips, support the upper back and use a wall to rest the legs. This gentle inversion is an excellent way to soothe the general body discomfort often accompanying headaches. The pelvis and torso are lifted, while the shoulders and head are supported. The result is a slight lifting and opening of the chest.

To prepare, place the bolster long-side against the wall. Position a single-fold blanket perpendicular to the midpoint of the bolster. Have a rolled towel ready for your neck and an eye bag to relax the eyes.

Sit on the bolster with your legs parallel to the wall and bring your right arm and shoulder to the blanket. Roll onto your back and simultaneously swing your legs up the wall so that the back of your thighs are against the wall. The sitting bones should be as close to the wall as comfortable. Tight hamstrings require more space between the wall and the body. If there is any discomfort, lift the hips and rearrange the support until the buttocks, hips and pelvis are completely at ease.

Sense the legs hanging above the hips and allow the back of the heels to rest on the wall. Notice the upper back, shoulders and head. They should be resting on the folded blanket.

It is important that the neck is positioned to preserve its natural curve. If there is any strain or if the chin feels it is pressing into the chest, use a small rolled towel or neck pillow to support it. The prop should support (C7) the vertebra at the base of the neck near the shoulders, and not be placed in the center of the neck where the curve is the greatest.

Once the body has settled into the posture, place the eye bag over the eyes or secure the elastic band, if you are using one. Bring awareness into the breath. Let the breath flow to the tips of the toes and back to the crown of the head. Forget the external world for the next several minutes and do nothing. Doing nothing is a most important task for restoring balance and well-being to the body, mind and spirit.

Scan the body for any residue of tension; feel it dissolve into the pool created by the legs draining into the belly. Let the brain become tranquil, unclenching any lingering worries or fears. Notice the breath. As you inhale, observe the belly fill; and as you exhale, sense all the fatigue wash out of the body. Let the body ride the waves of the breath inviting the breath to deepen even more.

Enjoy the sensations of being inverted for up to 15 minutes. When ready, remove the eye bag, or head band, and bend your knees. Press the feet into the wall, lift the hips and push the bolster toward the wall as you slide your body away. Rest with your calves on the bolster, take a few slow even breaths and then roll to one side. Come up to a seated position slowly and notice how the body/mind feels.

5) Supported Reclining Pose

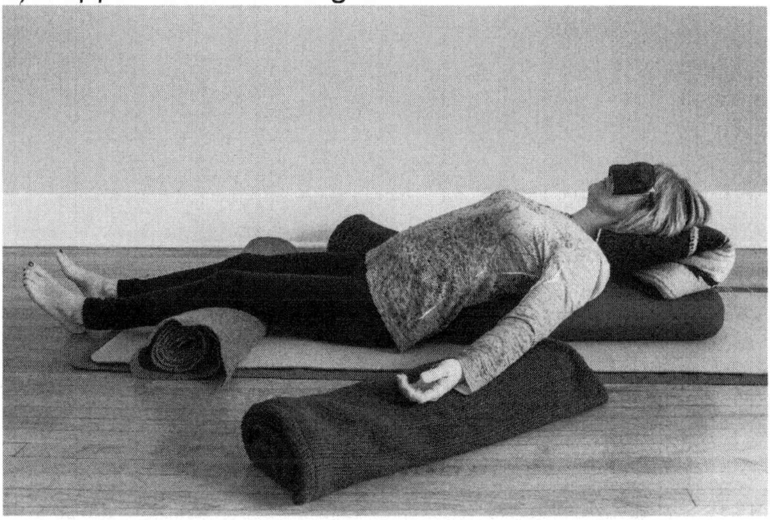

Props:

- Bolster
- Zafu
- 2 rolled blankets
- 1 or more folded blanket or towel
- Eye bag

Time:

- 10 minutes

Benefits:

- Helps with lung congestion
- Relieves tension between the shoulder blades
- Supports the kidneys

Cautions:

If you have any discomfort in the lower back, rearrange the props.

If after your practice, there is discomfort in your lower back, do not stay in this pose as long next time.

Supported Reclining Pose is a favorite because the props create the feeling you are resting in a chaise lounge somewhere far away from all frustrations and worries. It's like a mini-vacation. While reclining, let your imagination take you to your favorite vacation spot.

Place a bolster on the floor, short end at your lower back, and add a folded blanket to the other end to support your head. Have a zafu or rolled blanket ready to slide under your knees. Two additional blankets rolled long ways can be positioned on either side of your body for each forearm. Supporting your elbow and arm in this way relieves carpel tunnel, as well as discomfort in the neck and shoulders. With the props in place, bend your knees, slide the zafu under them and lean back onto the bolster. Your feet should rest softly on the floor with the legs naturally rolling out. Secure the head wrap, if using one or place an eye bag over your eyes, and feel the arms drape over their supports.

As you settle into the props, notice how the body feels. It is important to have your head and chest higher than your belly. Do not allow your chest to collapse. If there is any discomfort, make whatever adjustments necessary to let go completely. Come into the breath and watch the body as it finds its own natural, effortless rhythm. Body sensations will lead you deeper into that inner landscape.

Swallow and relax your throat and jaw. Let the cheekbones soften and feel the tongue float inside the mouth. Allow the forehead to melt and the eyebrows to soften. As you exhale, feel your body soften deep into the pelvis. Sense all tension draining away as you continue to breathe long, slow, even, effortless breaths.

As the physical body releases, mental and emotional tensions may arise. If so, allow them to be there, even welcome them. Without judging, notice what arises in each moment and give each sensation space to expand and dissolve. Often our tension simply wants to be noticed. When ready to return to waking consciousness, slowly move the body coming into an upright seated position. Take your calm, relaxed state of mind with you for the rest of your day.

Life
brings cycles
of activity and rest.

We
need both
to find balance,
health and well-being.

Rest
brings a time to
renew, restore, and rejuvenate.

Chapter 7

Improve Your Sleep

In the moments before sleep
there is an instant when
surrender is complete.
~Danna Faulds

Disturbances in sleep patterns are common in our culture and often come from unnecessary body tension and unhealthy patterns of thinking. The poses in this series help soothe your senses, assist you in falling asleep with ease, and contribute to remaining asleep throughout the night.

Four poses have been chosen: *Supported Goddess Pose* to begin relaxing; *Supported Wide-Angle Pose* to quiet the mind; *Tranquility Pose* to reduce fatigue; and *Supported Reclining Pose* to bring overall comfort and deep rest. Regular practice of these poses prior to bedtime will break the poor sleep habits and provide an avenue for new healthy patterns to develop.

In Restorative Yoga, the practice of letting go is as important as the physical position of the body. You systematically move awareness through the body as the breath discovers places where tension is being held. The combination of the breath and a deep awareness of sensations draws you into the inner space of your being, allowing the healing process to begin.

Remember, as thoughts arise and fall away, you are simply the observer. Return to the vast space inside your body and rest in the stillness of your inner landscape.

(1) Supported Goddess Pose

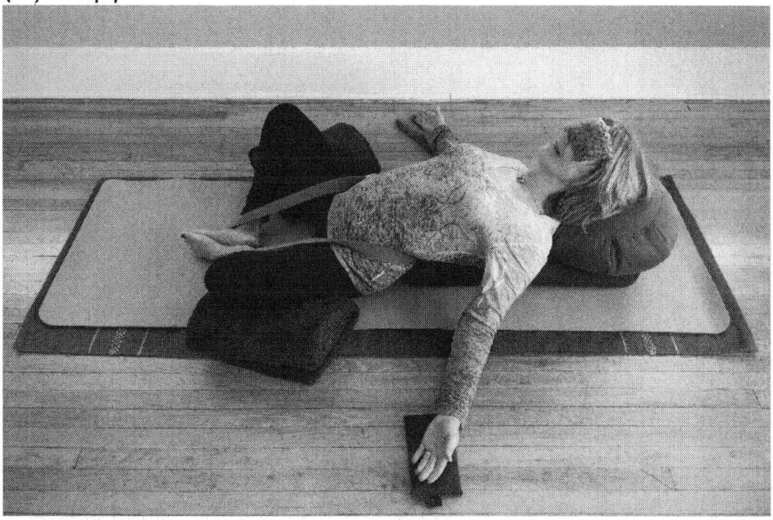

Props:

- Bolster
- Zafu
- 2 blankets or soft pillows
- Eye bag
- Belt or strap

Time:

- 7-10 minutes

Benefits:

- Helps balance blood pressure
- Improves circulation and respiration
- Relieves headaches
- Frees abdominal and pelvic restrictions

Cautions:

If you feel stiff after this pose, practice less the next time.

Supported Goddess or *Cobbler Pose* is considered one of the most important restorative poses. The props create a cradle in which the whole body receives nurturing as you snuggle into a deep sense of well-being and rest.

Preparing for this pose takes time, patience and several props: a bolster, two pillows, a zafu or two, an eye bag and maybe a blanket. Sit in front of the short end of the bolster with the tailbone touching it. Bring the soles of your feet together and allow your knees to open, as in *Cobbler Pose*.

Place a pillow or rolled blanket under each thigh so the legs and hips are totally supported. Even if you are supple and can open easily in cobbler, you need to support the weight of your legs. Care must be taken to avoid injuring or even straining the ligaments connecting the hips to the spine. The objective is to open the chest and relax the belly, rather than overstretch the inner thighs.

Use your arms for support as you lower your torso onto the bolster. Place a zafu under your head to support it and your neck. Make certain your spine is comfortable and you are supporting the sacrum. (You may need another zafu or a pillow to support the spine.)

Pillows or a folded blanket may also be placed under each arm to enhance the feeling of letting go. This will also relieve any tension in the neck and arms and relax the shoulders. Make sure the head and neck are supported. The forehead should be higher than the breastbone, and breastbone higher than pubic bone. The final position has your torso at a 45-degree angle to the floor.

A strap, or rolled towel, may be placed around the feet to prevent them from sliding. Fasten the strap into a loop that will fit around the hips and feet when lying in the pose. Take the strap over your head and adjust it around the hips. Then wrap the free side around the feet, with soles together. This should simply hold the feet in place and allow them to relax without sliding. A rolled towel or blanket will serve the same purpose.

Place an eye bag over your eyes and prepare to move into a deep state of relaxation. Bring awareness into the breath and feel the flow of the breath as it enters the nostrils and moves deeply into the chest, expanding into the belly. As you exhale, feel the whole body soften. Focus your awareness inside the body and feel the inner space grow with each breath. Rest into the vast spaciousness inside the body. Let the body/mind float on the breath as it moves in and out slowly, smoothly and evenly.

Consider being held in this cradle for 7-10 minutes. After relaxing so deeply, allow the body/mind to return slowly. Move deliberately in order to have the deep sense of peace fill every fiber of your being. Gently straighten the legs and release any accumulated tension in the knees.

Supported Goddess Pose reduces fatigue, improves breathing and is helpful for those with high blood pressure, headaches, or digestive problems.

(2) Supported Wide-Angle Pose

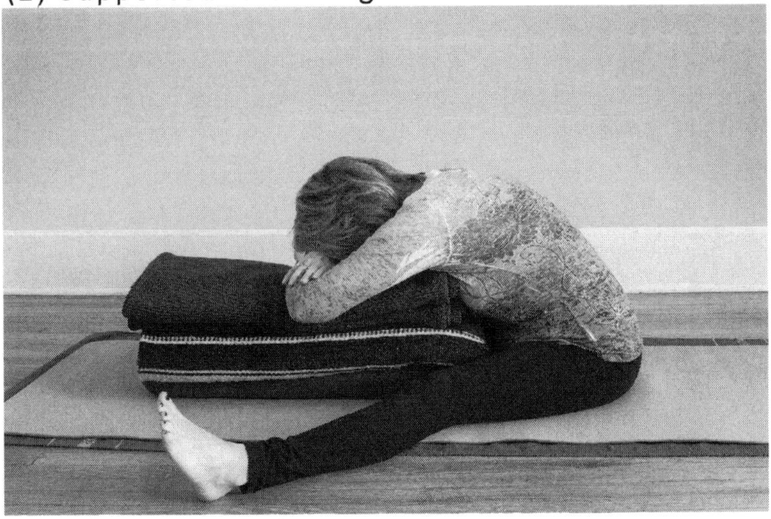

Props:

Bolster
1 or more folded blankets
Eye bag

Time:

1-6 minutes

Benefits:

Quiets organs of digestion and elimination
Opens the lower back
Provides space for the kidneys

Cautions:

Make sure your neck, lower back and knees are comfortable. If there is pain, do not remain in this pose.

Skip this pose if you have back pain, even after

adjusting the height of the props under your head and chest or those upon which you may be sitting.

With appropriate support, this variation of a seated forward bend enhances relaxation, calms the mind and quiets the internal organs. As you prepare this posture, be aware of all body sensations. If you find discomfort in your knees, inner thighs, or lower back, immediately make adjustments.

This is not a pose to stretch the legs or back. The purpose is to release mental and physical tension and to expand the back of the body. It has been reported to help relieve headaches which often interfere with sleep.

Bring a bolster between the legs as you sit on the floor. If the back of the legs are tight or your lower back rounds as you bend over the bolster, sit on the edge of a folded blanket to raise your pelvis and allow it to tilt forward slightly. Small rolled towels under each knee release tightness along the inner thighs.

Once you are comfortable, you have several options as to how you would like to rest. Your head could rest on folded arms or directly on the bolster. You may prefer to let your arms rest at your sides as the head nestles into the prop

Let your chin drop slightly, relaxing the throat and neck. Notice how you feel. If there is too much of a stretch, increase the height of the props by adding blocks or a blanket. If there is any discomfort, rest your head on the edge of a chair seat. (See the photo, p. 120)

If you find any unpleasant sensation in your lower back, even with these adjustments, you may have a condition that needs the attention of a health care provider. Please do not continue this or any pose in which you are experiencing pain.

If all is well, allow your body to be supported by the props. Notice your breath. As you inhale feel the inner body expand; and as you exhale feel the belly soften. Let your back shelter you from all external distractions. Feel every cell in your body surrender to the stillness within.

You might want to begin practicing this pose for a minute or two and increase to 5-6 minutes. As you sense your body is ready to come out of the pose, slowly move into a seated position using your arms to return upright. Place your hands behind you and lean back, open your eyes and breathe into the present moment.

Breathing
into the back body
brings attention to an often ignored
part of the body.

Yogis
believe the ego
is associated with the front of the body
while your deeper true nature is
found in the back body.

(3) Supported Tranquility Pose

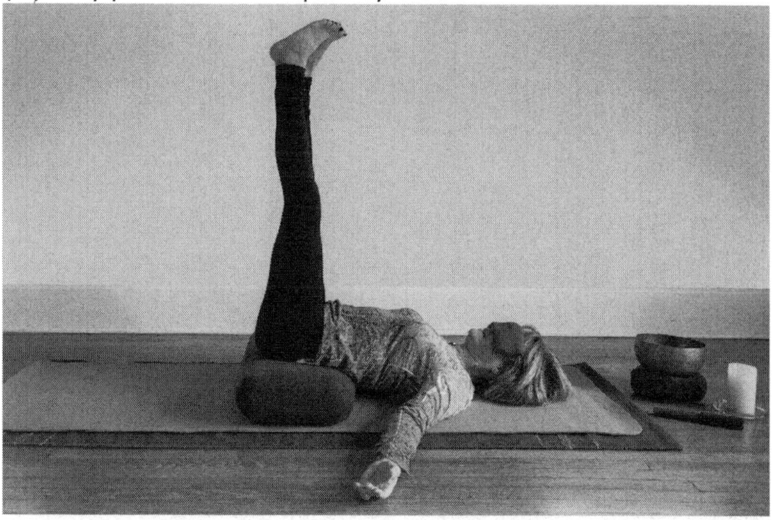

Props:

Bolster or zafu
1 or more folded blankets or towels
Eye bag

Time:

5-10 minutes

Benefits:

Restores tired legs and feet
Soothes the nervous system
Quiets the mind
Balances blood pressure
Regulates the thyroid gland

Cautions:

If your back is uncomfortable, bend your knees and place your feet on the floor, remove the cushion and move to the wall.

> Not recommended for those who should avoid inversions (hiatal hernia, eye pressure, retinal problems, heart condition, neck injury or are menstruating).
>
> If this pose creates pressure in the head, do not do it.

In this variation of *Tranquility Pose* the hips are elevated with a support and the leg bones nestle into the hip sockets. A favorite of students, this gentle inversion is a very effective way to relieve overall body discomfort. The pelvis and torso are lifted, while the shoulders and head are supported. The result is a slight lifting and opening of the chest.

To prepare for this pose, lie on your back with knees bent and feet close to the hips. Press your feet into the floor allowing the hips to lift. Slide a zafu or bolster under the hips and let them sink into the support. If there is any discomfort, lift the hips and rearrange the support until the buttocks, hips and pelvis are completely at ease.

Feel the legs reach slowly upward until they are hanging in the air above the hips. It is important they are directly above the hips in order for gravity to draw the top of the leg gently into the hip socket. The perfect placement is found when the legs can simply rest in the air without muscular tension. The weight of the leg releases both the hip joint and the low back.

If it is difficult to maintain the position, try the pose against the wall. With the wall supporting the legs, any need for holding them in the air vanishes. To assume this variation, move to a wall and sit with the right side of the body against the wall. Place a support next to the left hip.

Lie down on the floor and swing the legs up onto the wall. The sitting bones should be as close to the wall as comfortable. More space may be needed between the wall and the body if the hamstrings are tight.

Once the legs are on the wall, bend the knees and press the soles of the feet onto the wall to elevate the hips. Slide the cushion under and rest into the support. Make adjustments to be comfortable.

It is important that the neck is positioned to preserve its natural curve. If there is any strain or if the chin is pressing into the chest, use a small rolled towel or neck pillow to support it. The prop should support the vertebra at the base of the neck near the shoulders (C7), and not be placed in the center of the neck where the curve is the greatest.

Once the body has settled into the posture, place an eye bag over your eyes and bring awareness into the breath. Let the breath flow to the tips of the toes and back to the crown of the head. Forget the external world for the next several minutes and do nothing. Doing nothing aids in moving into stillness and preparing for a deep, restful sleep.

Scan the body for any residue of tension; feel it dissolve into the serene pool created by the legs draining into the belly. Let the brain become tranquil, unclenching any worries or fears that may linger. As you inhale, observe the belly fill and, as you exhale, feel all the fatigue wash out of the body. Let the body ride the waves of the breath inviting it to deepen even more.

Come into an awareness of the slight pause at the end of the exhalation and again at the end of inhalation. In this brief moment of stillness, feel the tranquility and deep rest of utter silence. Each breath bringing a stillness, a moment of just being.

Enjoy the sensations of being inverted for up to 15 minutes. When ready, remove the eye bag and bend your knees. Press the feet into the floor or the wall, as appropriate, and lift the hips just enough to remove the bolster. Slowly bring the hips back to the floor and roll to one side resting with the calves on the bolster. Take a few slow even breaths and then prepare to sit up. Remember to use your arms to lift the torso so that you do not strain your lower back. Come up to a seated position slowly and notice how the body/mind feels.

One of the greatest benefits of this pose is that it serves as an antidote for the systemic effects of stress. The slight inversion allows the mind to become tranquil. Regular practice brings relief to tired feet and legs and is especially beneficial to those with varicose veins. It may help establish new patterns for better sleep.

(4) Supported Reclining Pose

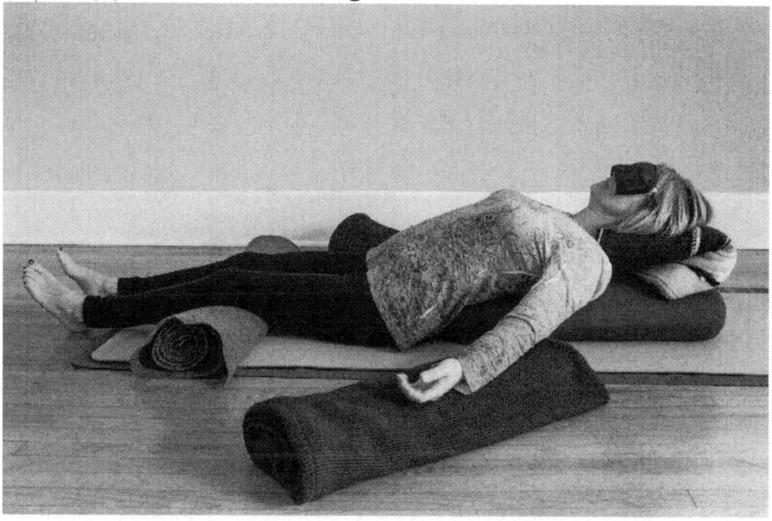

Props:

- Bolster
- Zafu
- 2 rolled blankets
- 1 or more folded blankets or towels
- Eye bag

Time:

- 10 minutes

Benefits:

- Helps with lung congestion
- Relieves tension between the shoulder blades
- Supports the kidneys

Cautions:

It is important to have your head and chest higher than your belly and do not collapse your chest.

> If after your practice, there is discomfort in your lower back, do not stay in this pose as long next time.

Supported Reclining Pose is perfect as an antidote for trouble sleeping because it calms the nervous system which allows your sleep pattern to change. The props create the feeling you are resting in a chaise lounge somewhere far away from all worries, concerns and frustrations. It's like a mini-vacation. Let your imagination take you to your favorite vacation spot.

A good night's sleep can become a habit when tension is relieved. Tension builds in various places due to habits of thinking, belief systems, and body posture. These habits reinforce the tension turning it into chronic pain or recurring discomfort. Taking time to undo these habits can be as simple as practicing this enjoyable pose.

Place a bolster on the floor, short end at your lower back, and add a folded blanket to the other end to support your head. Have a zafu or rolled blanket ready to slide under your knees. Two additional blankets folded long ways can be positioned on either side of your body for each forearm. Supporting your elbow and arm in this way relieves carpel tunnel, as well as discomfort in the neck and shoulders. With the props in place, bend your knees, slide the zafu under them and lean back onto the bolster. Your heels should rest softly on the floor, legs naturally rolling out. Place an eye bag over your eyes, and feel the arms drape over their supports.

As you settle into the props, notice how the body feels. It is important to have your head and chest higher than your belly. Do not allow your chest to collapse. If there is any discomfort, make the necessary adjustments to let go completely. Come into the breath and watch the body as it finds its own natural, effortless rhythm. Body sensations will lead you deeper into your inner landscape.

Swallow and relax your throat and jaw. Let the cheekbones soften and the tongue float inside the mouth. Feel the forehead melt and the eyebrows soften. As you exhale, let a soft sigh escape from your lips as your belly drops deep into the pelvis. Sense all tension draining away as you continue to breathe long, slow, even, and effortless breaths.

As tension in the physical body releases, mental and emotional tensions may arise. If so, allow them to be there, even welcome them. No judging, just notice what arises in each moment and give each sensation space to expand and dissolve. Often our discomfort simply wants to be noticed.

After ten minutes or longer allow your awareness to return. Bend your knees and push the zafu away with your feet. Roll to one side and take a few breaths. Move slowly, remove your eye bag and allow your eyes to adjust to the light.

When you feel ready, resume your evening preparations for sleep and enjoy a good night's sleep.

When you find a position
so comfortable that your body is light and open
and your breath is soft and quiet,
you have reached an experiential understanding of
Restorative Yoga.

You have made the practice your own.
You no longer "do,"
but rather simply
"be."

Chapter 8

Rejuvenate From Exhaustion

You have traveled too fast over false ground;
Now your soul has come to take you back.
Take refuge in your senses, open up
To all the small miracles you rushed through.
~John O'Donohue

Our busy lives frequently bring feelings of exhaustion. This is particularly true after traveling, recovering from an extended illness, long-term care giving, or overcoming a difficult loss. All these circumstances are the perfect time to return to or to begin a Restorative Yoga practice.

Exhaustion may come in many forms, but it always requires time to restore your natural vitality and well-being. Proper nutrition, adequate rest and exercise are important components to reviving your health. In addition, restorative poses regularly practiced bring a deep sense of serenity and balance to your life.

The poses in this final series can be practiced anywhere. If traveling, props can be fashioned from blankets, towels and pillows found in hotel rooms. You can find a small space in your luggage to tuck an eye bag.

Just knowing you are able to access these postures anywhere, brings assurance that comfort, peace and relief from tension are available when needed.

Four poses are included here: *Legs Up the Wall Pose, Supported Bridge Pose, Supported Wide-Angle Pose,* and *Shavasana Pose with Legs Elevated.* These postures offer the opportunity to rest in gentle inversions, a calming forward bend, and the premier resting pose with your legs lifted on cushions. Together they bring balance and time to rejuvenate.

1) Legs Up the Wall Pose

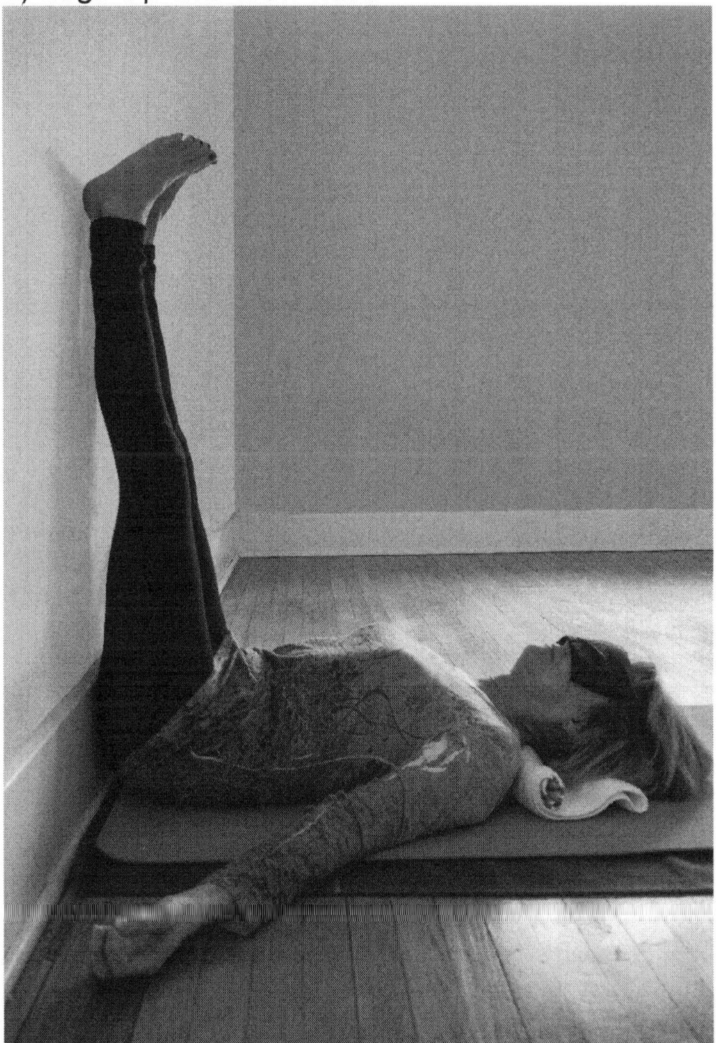

Props:

- An extra mat (optional)
- 1 or more folded blankets or towels
- Eye bag

Time:

5-10 minutes

Benefits:

Restores tired legs and feet
Soothes the nervous system
Quiets the mind
Relieves headaches
Balances blood pressure
Regulates the thyroid gland

Cautions:

Not recommended for those who should avoid inversions, if you have a hiatal hernia, eye pressure, retinal problems, heart condition, neck injury or are menstruating.

Legs Up the Wall Pose is a variation of *Tranquility Pose* in which the floor supports your back and a wall supports the legs. This gentle inversion is a very effective way to relieve the overall body discomfort often accompanying exhaustion. The pelvis, torso, shoulders and head are supported by the mat and the floor.

Place your mat along with a single-fold blanket perpendicular to the wall. Have a small rolled towel ready for your neck and an eye bag to soothe the eyes.

Sit at the edge of the mat with one shoulder next to the wall. Roll onto your back and simultaneously swing your legs up the wall so that the back of your thighs are against the wall. The sitting bones should be as close to the wall as comfortable. Tight hamstrings will require more space between the wall and the body. If there is any discomfort, move your torso away from the wall. The buttocks, hips and pelvis should be completely at ease.

Sense the legs hanging above the hips and allow the back of the heels to rest on the wall. Now, notice the upper back, shoulders and head. They should be resting on the folded blanket.

The natural curve of the neck needs to be maintained. Use a small rolled towel or pillow to support the neck if there is any strain or if the chin presses into the chest. The prop should support (C7) the vertebra at the base of the neck near the shoulders, and not be placed in the center of the neck where the curve is the greatest.

Place the eye bag over your eyes and bring awareness into the breath. Let the breath flow to the tips of the toes and back to the crown of the head. Forget the external world for the next several minutes and do nothing. Doing nothing is a most important task for restoring balance and well-being to the body, mind and spirit.

Scan the body for any residue of tension; feel it dissolve as the legs drain into the belly. Let the brain become tranquil, unclenching any lingering worries or fears. Notice the breath; inhale observing the belly fill and exhale feeling all the fatigue wash out of the body. Let the body ride the waves of the breath inviting the breath to deepen even more.

Enjoy the sensations of being inverted for up to 15 minutes. When ready, remove the eye bag and bend your knees. Press your feet into the wall as you slide your body away from the wall. Rest in a curled position and take a few slow even breaths. Come up to a seated position slowly and notice how the body/mind feels.

Inverted poses, such as this one, are beneficial in relieving fatigue, particularly to people who sit or stand for prolonged periods of time. Moreover, postures that invert the legs allow gravity to act on the lymphatic system. This system is a vital part of the immune system and works to defend the body against infections. The improved circulation resulting from this gentle inversion offers a gentle, refreshing way to strengthen the immune system.

(2) Supported Bridge Pose

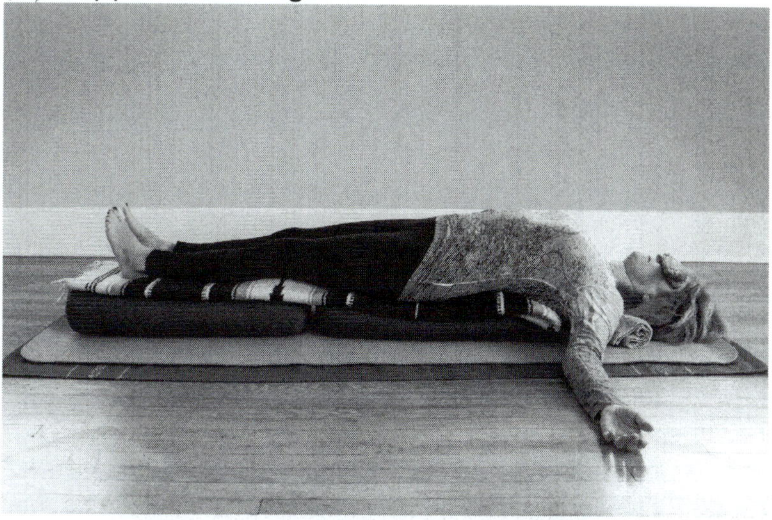

Props:

2 bolsters or 2 stacks of folded blankets
Eye bag

Time:

8-10 minutes

Benefits:

Reduces fatigue
Quiets the mind
Relieves discomfort of sitting too long
Opens the chest and releases shoulder tension
Drains fluid from the legs
Relieves soreness in hips and legs

Cautions:

Not recommended for those who need to avoid inversions (hiatal hernia, eye pressure, retinal problems, heart problems or neck problems).

Avoid if you have a respiratory or sinus infection.

This modified inversion, *Supported Bridge,* helps "bridge the gap" between past and future by connecting you to the present moment. Being present means you are aware of the sensations in your body/mind. Staying in your body is particularly helpful when you are exhausted, overworked, or fatigued from travel.

Place two bolsters, or stacks of blankets, end-to-end so that your entire torso and legs will fit on them. The shoulders, neck and head will be on the floor. The height of the props depends on the flexibility of your upper back. Most people are comfortable with props between 6-12 inches in height. You might want to start with blankets to determine how high the supports need to be. Also, make certain the height is uniform throughout the length of the prop.

Straddle the bolsters nearer to the end directly behind your head. Using the strength of your arms, lower your body to the props. Slide off the end so your head and shoulders touch the floor and you are looking at the ceiling. If your lower back has any discomfort, bend your knees and place your feet on the bolster or on the floor on either side of it.

If your chin is moving into your chest, you need to support the vertebra located at the base of your neck (C7), near the shoulders. You can use a rolled towel, washcloth or small pillow. Roll the towel enough to support this area. It is important not to have too much support in this area, just enough to release the chin.

Cover your eyes with the eye bag and begin to notice your breath. Make certain you are comfortable and let your arms rest slightly away from your sides. Feel the lungs and ribs expand with each inhale. Let your awareness move inward with each exhale.

Notice how the breath can lead you into that vast inner space where you can rest. Let the stillness and silence nurture and soothe your body, mind and spirit.

After 10-15 minutes or as long as you are comfortable, begin to come back. Let the eye bag slide off your face as your body slides in the direction of your head. Rest your lower legs on the bolster while your back releases into the floor. After several breaths, roll to one side and return to a seated position.

(3) Supported Wide-Angle Pose

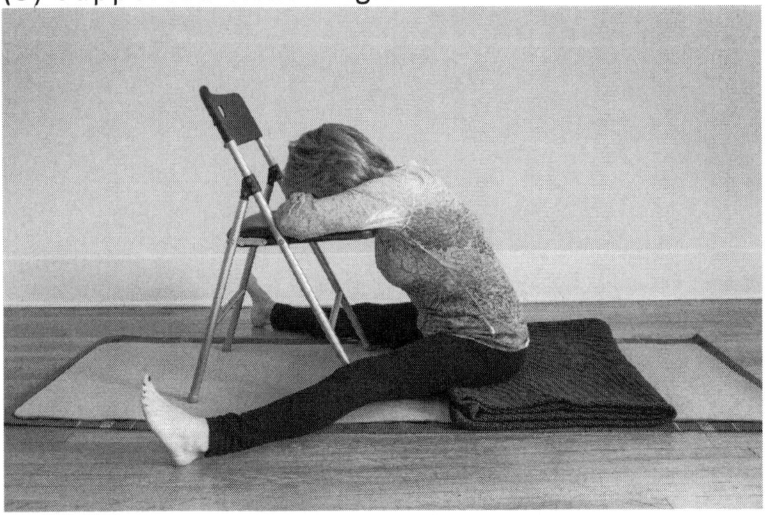

Props:

- Bolster
- 1 or more folded blankets
- Eye bag

Time:

- 1-6 minutes

Benefits:

- Quiets organs of digestion and elimination
- Opens the lower back
- Provides space for the kidneys

Cautions:

Make sure your neck, lower back and knees are comfortable. If there is pain, do not continue this pose.

With appropriate support, this variation of a seated forward bend enhances relaxation, calms the mind and quiets the internal organs. As you prepare this posture, be aware of all body sensations. If you find discomfort in your knees, inner thighs, or lower back, immediately make adjustments. If your back is still uncomfortable, skip this pose.

This is not a pose to stretch the legs or back, but rather the objective is to release mental and physical tension and to expand the back of the body.

The gentler version of this pose has you sit with your legs outstretched on either side of a folding chair. Make a "pillow" with your forearms and rest your head. If the back of the legs are tight or your lower back rounds as you move your torso toward the chair, use a folded blanket to lift and tilt your pelvis forward.

The other variation for this posture is to sit on the floor with your outstretched legs separated in a "v." and allow your torso to move toward the support. (See photo, p. 100). If the back of the legs are tight or your lower back rounds as you bend over the bolster, sit on the edge of a folded blanket to raise your pelvis and allow it to tilt forward slightly. Small rolled towels under each knee release tightness along the inner thighs.

Once you are comfortable, you have several options as to how you would like to rest. Your head could rest on folded arms or directly on the bolster or chair. You may prefer to let your arms rest at your sides as the head nestles into the prop.

Whichever variation you choose, let your chin drop slightly, relaxing the throat and neck. Notice how you feel. If there is too much of a stretch, increase the height of the props (or chair seat) by adding a blanket.

If you find any unpleasant sensation in your lower

back, even with these adjustments, you may need the attention of a health care provider. Please do not continue this, or any pose, in which you are experiencing pain.

Let go and allow your body to be supported by the props. Notice your breath. As you inhale feel the inner body expand; as you exhale feel the belly soften. Let your back shelter you from all external distractions. Feel every cell in your body surrender to the stillness within.

You might want to begin practicing this pose for a minute or two and increase to 5-6 minutes. As you sense when your body is ready to come out of the pose, slowly move into a seated position using your arms to return upright. Place your hands behind you and lean back, open your eyes and breathe into the present moment.

(4) Shavasana Pose with Legs Elevated

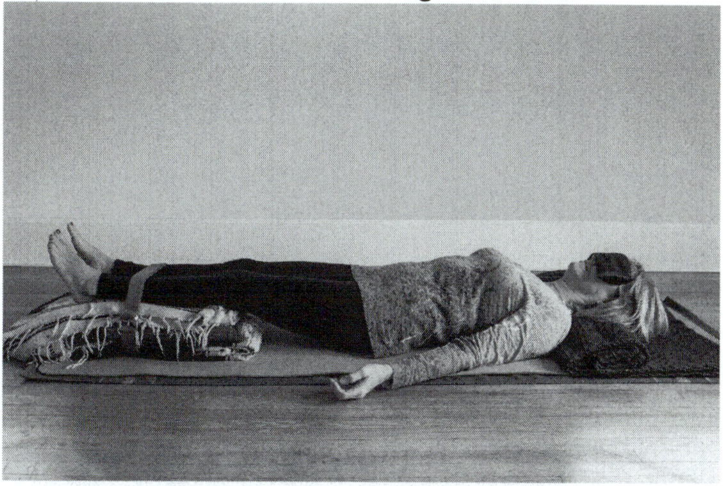

Props:

3 or more folded blankets
Eye bag
Strap or Belt
Sand bag, optional

Time:

10-15 minutes

Benefits:

Reduces fatigue, stress and anxiety
Lowers blood pressure and heart rate
Enhances immune system
Quiets the mind

Cautions:

Practice a side-lying variation of this pose if you are more than three months pregnant.

Shavasana, or Corpse Pose, places the least metabolic demand on your body of any pose. Practicing this posture is one of the best things you can do for yourself. It provides the space for recovering from exhaustion.

For this variation of *Shavasana Pose,* you need three or more folded blankets to create a stack about a foot high. You may want to cover yourself during this pose because your body temperature will drop as your relaxation deepens. Have another blanket at the other end of the mat. Roll one end of it three or four times to make a support for your neck. The back of your head rests on the unrolled portion of the blanket.

Come onto your mat with the stack of blankets at the end where your feet are. Bring the calves to rest on the blankets. Wrap a Yoga belt or strap around the legs and blankets to keep them secure. Check to see that your chin is slightly lower than your forehead as you rest on the blanket. This chin position signals the brain to relax. Cover your eyes with an eye bag and let your arms rest just far enough from your body to release all tension.

Let the floor support you as you unwind. Remember, there is nowhere to go and nothing to do. Breathe long, slow, even breaths. Turn inward and find the vast spaciousness inside the body. Rest for as long as you would like, 10-15 minutes.

Begin to come back by releasing the strap and slowly bending one knee and then the other. Feel the body move to one side as your eye bag slides off the eyes. Rest in a fetal position for a few breaths before coming back to a seated position. Remember to use your hands and the strength of your arms to come up. Notice how you feel and take your time as you continue through your day.

Chapter 9

Restorative Living

Let your practice unfold from inside.
Think of it as a silk thread, smooth and strong.
Let it connect you to the stillness found within.
~ Nancy Hodge Long

Establishing Your Practice

Now that there is a framework, let's find a way to establish a practice. Many students find it difficult to initiate an on-going practice even though they know they will feel better.

Here are some suggestions for getting started:

1) Find a quiet place to practice where you won't be disturbed.
2) Decide how long you would like to practice and choose poses that will meet your needs.
3) Gather the necessary props.
4) Select quiet music to complement your practice, if you wish.
5) Roll out your mat and lie on the floor.

6) Take a few minutes to tune into the sensations in your body and to recognize where tension is being held.
7) Let the breath be your guide to deep awareness of the body/mind in the present moment.
8) Be open to whatever arises in each moment without trying to control or manipulate.
9) Let each pose unfold effortlessly.

Your practice is a unique experience reflecting the conditions associated with the state of your body, mind, and emotions, as well as the environment.

There may be times practice brings a sense of calm and quiet. Other times you may find yourself recharged and energized. Remember, your practice can be formal or informal, long or short, focused or relaxed.

Formal practice includes a sequence of poses designed for a specific outcome: releasing tension or stress, relieving chronic pain, improving sleep, or increasing flexibility in the spine. There may be a specific duration of time to remain in each pose, as well as a particular order to follow.

As you become familiar with Restorative Yoga, the poses, or series of poses, that are just right may come to mind effortlessly. The full practice offers a series of poses for the health of the overall spine. They engage the spine in its entire range of movement. This practice requires a block of time you may not have on a daily basis. In that case, you are free to choose two or three poses that feel right to you.

At first, any attempt to design your own practice may feel overwhelming. Each time you try, however, you will learn more about Yoga, the poses, and yourself.

When you do not have the appropriate space or enough time for a formal practice, a welcome substitute can be an informal practice. *Legs Up the Wall Pose* works wonders after a stressful day. Or perhaps you have a break at work and you choose to do *Half-Dog Pose* or *Supported Seated Forward Bend Pose* at your desk.

Remember to begin your practice by noticing the body/mind. Taking even a few minutes to move into a deep sense of the present moment will carry you to Yoga's door. This door is always open, ready to greet you with compassion and complete acceptance.

An essential element of your practice is the breath. Notice the breath. Feeling it move through the nostrils will bring the mind into a quiet space. Tuning into the breath is a necessary component to every practice.

The breath is a tool assisting you to stay present in each moment. Be the observer and notice how the body/mind responds to every pose. If at any time you feel pain or discomfort, move out of that position.

One day you may feel so fatigued you can barely move. Take just 10-15 minutes to practice *Supported Tranquility Pose*. This pose brings a state of calm while allowing gravity to reverse its effects on the body. The benefits of even a few minutes in this position are truly amazing.

Supported Goddess (or Cobbler) Pose is a favorite of many students. It is their "go-to" pose after a stressful day. It relieves anxiety and brings a deep sense of safety and protection.

Always take a few minutes at the end to return to *Shavasana*. It is important to integrate the experience each time you practice. If you are doing a brief, informal practice, be creative and find a way to relax completely before returning to your day's activities.

You may wish to keep a journal of your practice. This provides a record of the poses and how they affect you. You could simply mark the pages in this book so you can easily turn to the pose and remember how to practice it.

Finding Balance

Finding balance in your life is essential for your health and well-being. There are many things you can do to bring balance into your everyday living. First, you need to be aware of how your activities are affecting you. Taking time to recognize what your body needs in a given moment can help with this. The idea of finding balance is truly an expression of the innate flexibility that Yoga offers.

Once you recognize your needs, determine a way to meet them. Establish a regular time for self-care. Besides practicing Yoga, you may want to schedule a massage or facial, time for tea or coffee with a close friend, a walk in nature, or time to just be.

The practice of Yoga is not an athlete's discipline of rigid structure and striving. Rather it offers a lifeline to your essence. It is a way to return to your Self each time you feel something is amiss. If you are hesitant about your practice, remember the only bad practice is the one you did not do. There is no right or wrong and no place for judgment.

Many love the morning and begin each day with the desire to practice. Others find the evening is best. Some days, time in the morning or evening is easy to find. Other days your schedule is too full for anything more than an informal modified *Child's Pose* at your desk or *Half-Dog Pose* at the kitchen counter before dinner preparations begin.

For many students, *Supported Goddess Pose* feels like being held in the womb of the universe. In a place so vast and welcoming, you are truly bathed in unconditional love, total acceptance and genuine compassion. This pose can restore your personal power bringing courage and inner strength. It reminds you that everything in the universe is perfect just as it is.

Supported Bridge Pose is a gentle backbend and a slight inversion. It brings the mind into a place of balance. It brings a deep "letting go" of all worries and frustrations, fears and concerns. The backbend allows your body to open deeply through the thoracic spine and ribcage. This supports respiration and gives the lungs a chance to breathe without restrictions caused by poor posture, a defeated attitude or that favorite chair.

Whatever poses feel right are the ones you need to do. If you think you would like to do *Child's Pose* and there is no relief, you need to come out of it and try something else. It may take time to become familiar enough with the poses to be able to discern which might work at a particular time. It is better for you to feel your way into a practice than to follow mindlessly without connecting the pose to how your body/mind is responding.

Embracing Each Moment

Living in a way that restores and rejuvenates you is a practical and resourceful way to live. One of the first things Yoga teaches is to be aware of the body/mind in each moment. It is amazing how often you move through your day oblivious to what is happening. Staying embodied anchors you to the present moment, to what is real. Whenever you use your senses to notice how you feel, you are practicing awareness of the body/mind.

For instance, the mind can be preoccupied with a future event or ruminating about some past action. These thoughts may be pleasant or unpleasant. Either way they draw us out of the present moment; but just noticing the mind has wandered off is enough to bring you back to whatever sensations are present in the body/mind. Now you are back in the present moment. This is the only thing that is real. Even thoughts and memories occur in the present moment. This moment is all you truly have.

Part of embracing each moment is the recognition that you are responsible for how you view your life. Once you begin to observe yourself in each moment, you may discover there is a voice in your mind telling you what's right and wrong. This voice can be full of harsh criticism and self-judgment. Just because you hear this voice, you can choose to listen or just let it be without attaching to it.

Soothing poses are beneficial as you practice staying in the present moment. *Supported Child's Pose* brings comfort and the feeling of safety and security. The breath is directed into the back body where the spine can stretch, lengthen and release. The muscles of the back can form a gentle comforter allowing you to feel protected as the world dissolves and the body melts into the supports.

Supported Fish Pose expands the chest and releases the muscles of the upper back. Emotionally, this pose opens the heart space and allows you to find comfort and compassion for yourself. You might feel old wounds or traumas surface. Try to just be with whatever sensations arise. Once you welcome them into your heart space, they can find completion and dissolve.

Even when the present moment brings unwanted challenges or obstacles, Yoga teaches us to be with whatever is unfolding. Embracing each moment does not mean we must passively accept pain or discomfort. Instead, become the witness and simply observe the thoughts, emotions, images and sensations knowing they will come and go.

Remember you always have a choice to let go or remain attached. Everything in life changes, so it is good to learn to stay alive and alert in each moment. The Yoga Sutra teaches that holding on when it is time to let go will bring suffering. Often our pain lies in our inability to move on when it is clearly time to do so. Embracing each moment offers the chance to be fully alive and clearly present.

Learning to Love Yourself

For many, it is not easy to let go of self-judgment but learning to accept yourself in each moment is a primary lesson of Yoga. The ancient Yogis tell us that you cannot accept others without judgment if you do not first accept yourself. Before you can love another, you must learn to love yourself, just as you are.

Pema Chodron, American Buddhist nun and author of many books, explains we must first learn to be honest, loving, and compassionate toward ourselves before we can cultivate loving-kindness. There is great relief and a sense of freedom when you accept all of the parts of yourself and truly begin to love who you are.

Cultivate compassion for yourself by spending time alone in silence. Being comfortable with silence develops as you learn to be in the present moment without expecting any particular outcome and accepting each moment just as it is. This may seem difficult to do, but try it. You may find yourself relaxing into life as if it were an easy chair, made to fit you perfectly.

Often when you do not like someone or judge him/her, what is actually happening is something in you is being reflected in his/her words or actions. Observing interactions with others helps you consider the situation from their perspective. Recognizing life provides everyone with struggles, strengths and weaknesses, compassion for others can begin to blossom.

One of the most nurturing of the restorative poses is *Supported Goddess Pose*. The props in this pose create a space in which the body/mind can surrender and let the universe hold you. A sense of being loved and protected can be felt in this posture.

Supported Child's Pose offers a space to feel protected and sheltered from the troubles of the world. In this space compassion and love of self can blossom into an authentic sense of loving-kindness for all other beings.

Read Something Inspirational Each Day

So many books, ancient and new, offer spiritual insights and uplifting reminders to bring you back to the recognition that your true nature is an unchanging essence, a spark of the divine. Being in the light of those who have traveled before us, we are strengthened, encouraged, and supported as we experience each moment of our life.

Whatever your belief system, you can discover the beauty of life expressed through a variety of spiritual texts. This ancient wisdom has been read and loved for centuries in many different forms. Reading from these sacred books offers comfort and insight. We are bombarded with so many negative messages about our world, but we can counterbalance this by exposing ourselves to spiritual writing from the great mystics of all religions.

Contrary to Western culture's idea of Yoga as a fitness practice, traditional Yoga, as codified by Patanjali more than two thousand years ago, is a much more complex system. His definitive text, *The Yoga Sutra,* consists of 195 concise statements (sutras) explaining the deeper, essential aspects of Yoga theory and practice. Numerous translations are available and serious Yoga students engage in a lifelong study of this text.

Patanjali presents Yoga as having eight limbs. It is known as Raja yoga, or the royal path, because the eight limbs can lead to the full realization of your true self or inner nature. According to T. K. V. Desikachar in *The Heart of Yoga,* these eight limbs "develop concurrently and in an interrelated way." (p. 107) The royal path engages the body/mind in order to still the fluctuations of the mind. The *Yoga Sutra* states this stilling of the mind allows the light of your true spirit to shine.

The eight limbs are: Yamas, Niyamas, Asana, Pranayama, Pratyahara, Dhrana, Dhyana, and Samadhi. The first five limbs are external and relate to practices associated with your body, energy, senses, and the way you interact with the world. The remaining three are internal or mental limbs and offer practices to reveal your true nature.

It is not enough to engage in Asana (practice the poses) without considering Pranayama (the breath) or the other deeper aspects. All eight limbs are necessary, combining together to create a complete system.

The Yamas and Niyamas offer attitudes and moral precepts. Yamas describe the attitudes you have toward things and other people and ethical strategies to guide you. Niyamas are the ways you relate to yourself inwardly and provide insight into your habits and behavior patterns.

One of the Niyamas directly related to reading inspirational literature is Svadhyaya. Svadyaya is defined as self-study and includes observing yourself through introspection and self-realization. Pondering your emotions, thoughts, actions and reactions serves to bring awareness of your deeper self and your true nature. This Niyama also encourages you to read the ancient texts. Desikachar explains that you need reference points as you practice self-examination. The Yoga Sutra says you "will gradually find a link with the divine laws." (p.102)

The study of Yoga is a lifelong pursuit. Just this brief discussion is an indication of its depth and expanse. That is why as you establish a practice, Svadyaya is so important. Find a sacred book you are interested in studying and begin.

Before going to sleep is a powerful time to affect the subconscious mind. Taking 30 minutes to read from a book that nourishes your spirit will provide the space to rest deeply within your innermost space.

Spend Time with Like-Minded People

You may have observed that some people seem to always lift your spirit, while others drain your energy. Developing life habits to support your health and well-bring includes connecting with those who nourish your spirit. As Ram Dass, author of *Be Here Now,* writes, we are all just walking each other home. Wouldn't you rather walk with those who encourage and love you?

Yoga, the physical practice, is a combination of asana, breath and concentration. It offers you a tool to move deeply inside and connect with you who are. When you do this, you may find you can connect with those people who are truly kindred spirits.

As these relationships develop, they become the lifeline to help you through tough times, the touchstones to remind you when you lose your way, and your greatest fans to applaud you when you succeed.

Many Yoga practitioners schedule time to be with others who are interested in the study and practice of Yoga. This nourishes your spirit and provides encouragement to be consistent in your own practice. Time together can spark creative ways to incorporate the love of Yoga both on and off the mat. With a deeper understanding of Yoga and support of like-minded people, you can embrace the limitless possibilities of life.

Practice Each Day

The only "bad" practice is the one you don't do. Even if you only take a few minutes to stretch the spine in *Half-Dog Pose* or lie in *Shavasana,* it will make a difference.

Forming a habit of daily practice is like planting a seed and nurturing it so it will grow and blossom. If you plant the seed and then not tend it, it will wither and die. But consistent nurturing will bring it to fruition.

When your life is busy and you feel rushed in almost every moment, taking time to slow down is even more important. Habits can become like a tyrant ruling over us. The only thing to do is to start where you are.

Remember practice does not necessarily mean rolling out your mat and doing postures.

When old patterns begin to change into healthier habits of self-care, you will find life becomes easier and joy sprouts without effort. Take time to be in the present moment, just noticing your breath. Take time to truly listen to a friend or child. Notice your inner voice with compassion and respect. Just these simple things will provide the pathway to your personal practice.

If you do nothing else, take a few minutes for Shavasana each day. This one posture practiced consistently can change your life.

Let this practice of Restorative Yoga anchor you to your Self. Take precious moments to simply BE. Find ways to smile and share your smiles with everyone. Welcome each moment whether a joy or sorrow and discover the ground beneath that is always holding you. Open your heart and follow your own path.

Look within and find what you love.
Give yourself
the only gift you truly can
Awareness
in each moment.

Appendix

CHART OF PROPS

Prop	Description/Use	Substitute
Blanket	Firm, closely woven cotton or wool 62x80"	Large thick towels or firm quilts
Block 4x6x9"	Foam, wood, or cork	Stack of books
Bolster, Rectangular	Large, firm cushion	Firm pillow or sofa cushion – must provide support
Bolster, Round	Firm log-shaped cushion	Firm sofa cushions
Chair	Folding chair	Sturdy chair/no rollers
Elastic band	4" wide found in drugstores	Eye bag or man's silk tie
Eye bag	Silk or cotton 4"x8"x1"	Folded washcloth
Herbal Wraps	Various sizes, hot or cold	Folded towels
Mat	Nonskid, 24x68"	Any nonslip floor
Sandbag	10 lb. sturdy bag filled with sand	Bags of dried beans or rice
Strap	Cotton/D-ring 6, 8 or 10 feet long	Man's tie or wide tie (bathrobe)
Table	Stable, waist height & shoulder width	Add folded blankets or mats if needed
Wall	Flat, bare, no windows	Any vertical surface-higher than you
Zafu	Round cushion, filled with buckwheat hulls	Firm round cushion, large enough to sit on comfortably

INDEX OF POSES

ENDNOTES

Chapter 1

1. Donna Farhi, *Bringing Yoga to Life, The Everyday Practice of Enlightened Living* (San Francisco, CA: HarperCollins Publishers, 2003) p. 82.
2. Judith Hanson Lasater, Ph.D., P.T., (2013, September) *Experiential Anatomy.* Lisle, IL. Personal notes.
3. Nicholai Bachman, *The Yoga Sutras, An Essential Guide to the Heart of Yoga Philosophy* (Boulder, CO: Sounds True, Inc., 2010)
4. Richard Miller, Ph.D., *Yoga Nidra, the Meditative Heart of Yoga* (Boulder, CO: Sounds True, Inc., 2005)

Chapter 2

1. Danna Faulds, *From Root to Bloom, Yoga Poems and Other Writings* (Greenville, VA: Peaceable Kingdom Books, 2006) "Awareness Knowing Itself," p. 17.
2. Judith Hanson Lasater, Ph.D., P.T., *Relax and Renew: Restful Yoga for Stressful Times* (Berkeley, CA: Rodmell Press, 2011) p. 25.
3. Coleman Barks and Michael Green, *The Illuminated Prayer* (New York: Ballantine Books, 2000)
4. Richard Miller, Ph.D., *Breathing for Life, The Principles and Practice of Ujjayi Pranayama* (Sebastopol, CA: Anahata Press)

Chapter 3

1. Judith Hanson Lasater, Ph.D., P.T., *Relax and Renew: Restful Yoga for Stressful Times* (Berkeley, CA: Rodmell Press, 2011) pp. 33-34.
2. Richard Miller, Ph.D., *Savasana (Corpse Pose), Yoga*

Journal, November/December 1995

Chapter 4

1. Shih-Te, translated by Jerome Seaton, *Finding the Way Home: Awakening and Transformation* (Buffalo, NY: White Pine Press, 2010) p. 18.

Chapter 5

1. Richard Miller, Ph.D., *Breathing for Life, The Principles and Practice of Ujjayi Pranayama* (Sebastopol, CA: Anahata Press) p. 4.

Chapter 6

1. Robert Bly, translator, *Kabir Ecstatic Poems* (Boston, MA: Beacon Press, 1993) p. 19.

Chapter 7

1. Danna Faulds, *From Root to Bloom, Yoga Poems and Other Writings* (Greenville, VA: Peaceable Kingdom Books, 2006) "Whole and Weightless," p. 100.

Chapter 8

1. John O'Donohue, *To Bless the Space Between Us* (New York, NY: Doubleday, 2008) "For One Who Is Exhausted," p. 125.

Chapter 9

1. T.K.V. Desikachar, *The Heart of Yoga* (Rochester, VT: Inner Traditions International, 1999).
2. Ram Dass, *Be Here Now* (San Cristobal, NM: Lama Foundation, 1978).

BIBLIOGRAPHY

Nicholai Bachman, *The Yoga Sutras, An Essential Guide to the Heart of Yoga Philosophy* (Boulder, CO: Sounds True, Inc., 2010)

Coleman Barks and Michael Green, *The Illuminated Prayer* (New York: Ballantine Books, 2000)

Ram Dass, *Be Here Now,* (New York, NY: The Crown Publishing Group, 1978)

T.K.V. Desikachar, *The Heart of Yoga,* (Rochester, VT: Inner Traditions International, 1999)

Donna Farhi, *Bringing Yoga to Life, The Everyday Practice of Enlightened Living* (San Francisco, CA: HarperCollins Publishers, 2003)

Danna Faulds, *From Root to Bloom, Yoga Poems and Other Writings* (Greenville, VA: Peaceable Kingdom Books, 2006)

Judith Hanson Lasater, Ph.D., P.T., *Relax and Renew: Restful Yoga for Stressful Times,* (Berkeley, CA: Rodmell Press, 2011)

Richard Miller, PhD, *Yoga Nidra, the Meditative Heart of Yoga, (*Boulder, CO: Sounds True, Inc., 2005)

Michael Stone, *The Inner Tradition of Yoga: A Guide to Yoga Philosophy for the Contemporary Practitioner* (Boston, MA: Shambhala Publications, Inc., 2008)

Sandra Anderson and Rolf Sovik, Psy.D., *Yoga, Mastering the Basics,* (Honesdale, PA: The Himalayan Institute Press, 2000)

ABOUT THE AUTHOR

Nancy Hodge Long, MA, HITA, RYT, is a certified Yoga teacher with over 20 years' experience teaching Yoga and meditation. She studies with Judith Hansen Lasater, Richard Miller, Saul David Raye, Rod Stryker, and renowned master teachers from the Himalayan Institute. Her style weaves the ancient traditions of Hatha Yoga, Bhakti, and Tantra into a gentle, openhearted and authentic practice that welcomes all.

Nancy lives in Springfield, Illinois, with her husband, Michael, and their Golden Retriever, Bodhi. She offers Restorative Yoga, meditation and gentle Yoga practices to individuals and groups.

Nanyoga47@gmail.com
Facebook @ Timeless Gentle Yoga or Nancy Hodge Long
Website: www.timelessgentleyoga.com

37321746R00090

Printed in Great Britain
by Amazon